蜕变
METAMORPHOSIS
数字化种植导板与全瓷修复中的医技实践
CLINICAL AND TECHNOLOGICAL PRACTICES IN DIGITAL SURGICAL TEMPLATES AND CERAMIC RESTORATIONS FOR IMPLANTS

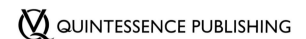

QUINTESSENCE PUBLISHING

Berlin | Chicago | Tokyo
Barcelona | London | Milan | Mexico City | Paris | Prague | Seoul | Warsaw
Beijing | Istanbul | Sao Paulo | Zagreb

余 涛
（Tao Yu）
刘海林 编著
（Hailin Liu）

METAMORPHOSIS
*Clinical and Technological Practices
in Digital Surgical Templates
and Ceramic Restorations
for Implants*

数字化种植导板
与全瓷修复中的医技实践

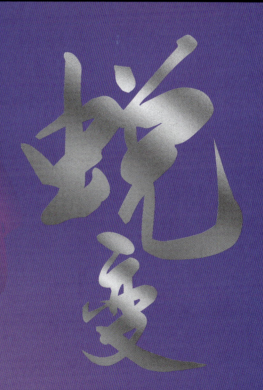

北方联合出版传媒（集团）股份有限公司
辽宁科学技术出版社

图文编辑

张　浩　刘玉卿　肖　艳　刘　菲　康　鹤　王静雅　纪凤薇　杨　洋　戴　军　张军林

图书在版编目（CIP）数据

蜕变：数字化种植导板与全瓷修复中的医技实践 / 余涛，刘海林编著. — 沈阳：辽宁科学技术出版社，2024.7
ISBN 978-7-5591-3630-5

Ⅰ . ①蜕… 　Ⅱ . ①余… ②刘… 　Ⅲ . ①数字技术—应用—种植牙—口腔外科学 　Ⅳ . ①R782.12-39

中国国家版本馆CIP数据核字（2024）第112327号

出版发行：辽宁科学技术出版社
　　　　　（地址：沈阳市和平区十一纬路25号　邮编：110003）
印 刷 者：凸版艺彩（东莞）印刷有限公司
经 销 者：各地新华书店
幅面尺寸：210mm×285mm
印　　张：17.5
插　　页：4
字　　数：350千字
出版时间：2024 年 7 月第 1 版
印刷时间：2024 年 7 月第 1 次印刷
出 品 人：陈　刚
责任编辑：殷　欣　苏　阳
封面设计：周　洁
版式设计：周　洁
责任校对：李　霞

书　　号：ISBN 978-7-5591-3630-5
定　　价：398.00 元

投稿热线：024-23280336
邮购热线：024-23280336
E-mail:cyclonechen@126.com
http://www.lnkj.com.cn

致敬口腔数字化变革中的每一分努力

To Every Effort in Evolution of Digital Dentistry

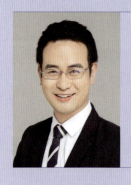

余 涛
Tao Yu

博士
DDS

北京大学口腔医学博士

瑞士日内瓦大学访问学者

北京大学口腔医院门诊部综合科主治医师

北京口腔医学会数字化口腔医学专业委员会委员

全国卫生产业企业管理协会数字化口腔产业分会学术秘书

国际数字化牙科学会（DDS）中国区委员、学术秘书

共同主编《口内数字印模技术》

参编《中国口腔数字化——从临床技术到病例精选》《美学区种植——从设计理念到临床实战》

《椅旁数字化修复实战——从入门到精通》《口腔数码摄影》等临床专著

Doctor Degree of Stomatology from School of Stomatology, Peking University

Visiting Scholar in Department of Fixed Prosthodontics and Biomaterials, University of Geneva, Switzerland

Attending Dentist in Department of General Dentistry, Clinical Division, Hospital of Stomatology, Peking University

Committee Member of Special Committee of Digital Dentistry, Beijing Stomatological Association

Academic Secretary of Chinese Society of Digital Dental Industry

Committee Member and Academic Secretary of Digital Dental Society (DDS) in China

Co-Editor-in-Chief of *Intraoral Digital Impression Technique*

Author of *Chinese Digital Dentistry - From Clinical Technology to Case Omnibus*, *Dental Implant in Esthetic Zone - From Design Concept to Clinical Practice*, *Practice of Chair-side Digitized Dental Restoration - From Beginner to Master*, and other a few dental clinical books

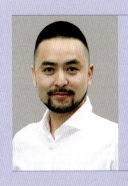

刘海林
Hailin Liu

牙科技师
Dental Technician

瑞佳义齿创始人
BPS®生物功能性义齿认证技师
The Dawson Academy毕业学员
全国卫生产业企业管理协会数字化口腔产业分会会员
主编《修复体制作精粹——种植上部修复》《蜕变——全牙列种植修复优化方案病例精选》
擅长领域：口腔摄影、BPS®生物功能性义齿、数字化种植及修复等

Ruijia Dentures-Founder
BPS® Biofunctional Denture Certified Technician
The Dawson Academy Graduation Internship
Member of Chinese Society of Digital Dental Industry
Editor-in-Chief of *The Essence of Restoration Production - Upper Implant Restoration, METAMORPHOSIS - Case Selection of the Optimal Plan for Full Arch Implantation and Restoration*
Expertise: dental photography, BPS® biofunctional dentures, digital implants and restorations

序一

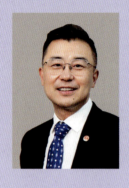

进入21世纪以来，数字化技术快速发展，给口腔临床诊疗方法带来了深刻的变革。大量低效率、高能耗、经验依赖的传统工作模式，已经向高效率、低能耗、可预测、可重复的新型数字化模式发展。

2013年，我们就预测在未来数字印模将逐渐成为主流；时至今日，中国的很多医疗机构已经在多数领域内用数字印模基本代替了传统物理印模，且数字印模的比例还在上升；静态导板、动态导航、手术机器人等数字化引导方式正在大范围地应用到临床，不断降低种植、牙周、根尖周等手术风险和难度；很多口腔义齿加工厂已经完成数字化转型或正在快速转型，使用各类先进数字化加工技术，将新型修复材料的性能发挥到极致，制造出功能与美学俱佳的修复体。

余涛医生是我们团队中非常优秀、勤奋的一员，我们一起工作了10余年，有幸见证了他在数字化口腔医学中的快速成长。他长期勤奋钻研数字化种植手术及数字化种植修复。从手术规划，到过渡修复体，再到永久修复体的设计与制作，他亲力亲为，积累了丰富的经验。通过分析大量病例，把对数字化种植和修复技术的总结编写成专著，这是他作为优秀临床医生和优秀教师责任感的充分体现，也将成为促进学科和专业发展、临床技术进步的新生力量。

刘海林技师专业技术过硬，在数字化技术领域有敏锐的眼光，深耕口腔数字化技术，尤其是数字化种植导板和数字化全瓷修复，数年以前就带领加工厂完成数字化转型。他完成并收集了大量成功的数字化病例资料，不断归纳、总结、提升、融入本书，供广大临床医生和技师参考。

口腔数字化技术的应用离不开良好的医技合作。余涛和刘海林这两位兢兢业业的口腔数字化实践者，紧密合作完成《蜕变——数字化种植导板与全瓷修复中的医技实践》一书，是更深层次的医技合作。本书从数字化导板、牙列缺损种植修复、全口种植修复、数字化修复材料等方面介绍相关理论知识和临床经验，并通过7个优秀病例，深入解析技术细节和难点。全书深入浅出、图文并茂，相信读者朋友们一定能找到共鸣、获得启发。

刘峰

北京大学口腔医院门诊部主任
北京大学口腔医院门诊部培训中心主任
全国卫生产业企业管理协会数字化口腔产业
分会会长
国际种植牙医师协会中国专家委员会副会长
中华口腔医学会口腔美学专业委员会常务委员
中华口腔医学会口腔种植专业委员会委员

Since the beginning of the 21st century, the rapid development of digital technology has profoundly transformed dental clinical diagnosis and treatment. Traditional working modes that were inefficient, high-energy-consuming, and experience-dependent have evolved into a new digital mode characterized by high efficiency, low energy consumption, predictability, and repeatability.

In 2013, we predicted that digital impressions would gradually become mainstream. Today, many dental hospitals and clinics in China have replaced traditional physical impressions with digital ones in most areas, and the proportion of digital impressions continues to grow. Digital guidance methods such as static templates, dynamic navigation, and surgical robots are widely applied in clinical practice, reducing the risks and difficulties of surgeries such as implant placement, periodontics, and periapical surgery. Many dental labs have completed or are rapidly undergoing digital transformation, utilizing various advanced digital processing technologies to maximize the performance of new restorative materials and produce functionally and aesthetically excellent restorations.

Dr. Tao Yu is an outstanding and diligent member of our team, with whom we have collaborated for more than ten years. It has been fortunate to witness his rapid growth in digital dentistry. He has long been dedicated to digital implant surgery and digital implant restoration. From surgical planning to transitional and permanent restorations, he has accumulated rich experience in every detail of planning, designing, and production. By analyzing numerous cases, he has summarized his experiences with digital implant placement and restoration techniques into a monograph. This work fully embodies his responsibility as an excellent clinician and educator at Peking University and will promote the development of the discipline and clinical technological advancements.

Technician Hailin Liu is highly professional with outstanding technical skills. He has a keen eye for digital technology, focusing deeply on digital dental technologies, especially digital guided surgical templates and digital all-ceramic restorations. Years ago, his dental lab transformed into a digital lab, where he has completed and collected many successful digital cases. He continuously summarizes and improves techniques, integrating them into this book for the reference of dentists and technicians.

The application of digital technology in dentistry relies on good cooperation between dentists and technicians. Tao and Hailin, two dedicated practitioners of digital dentistry, closely collaborated to compose the book *Metamorphosis – Clinical and Technological Practices in Digital Surgical Templates and Ceramic Restorations for Implants*. This book represents a deeper level of clinical and technical cooperation. It introduces relevant theoretical knowledge and clinical experience in areas such as digital templates, implant restorations for defective dentitions, full-arch implant restorations, and digital restoration materials. The book delves into technical details and challenges through seven outstanding cases. Presented in a comprehensive and illustrative manner, it is expected that readers will resonate with it and find inspiration.

Feng Liu

Director of Clinical Division, Hospital of Stomatology, Peking University
Director of the Training Center of Clinical Division, Hospital of Stomatology, Peking University
President of Chinese Society of Digital Dental Industry
Vice-President of Chinese Expert Committee of International Congress of Oral Implantologists
A standing committee member of Chinese Society of Esthetic Dentistry
A committee member of Chinese Society of Oral Implantology

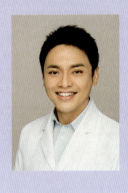

在口腔医学的快速发展中，数字化技术的引入为我们开辟了一个崭新的天地，尤其是在种植和修复领域的应用更是令人瞩目。作为一名口腔种植事业的耕耘者，我非常高兴看到余涛医生和刘海林技师携手编写的《蜕变——数字化种植导板与全瓷修复中的医技实践》一书，它将为广大口腔医生和技师带来重要的知识与实践指导。

种植手术的成功在很大程度上取决于种植体的精确植入，而数字化种植导板的出现正是为了实现这一目标。我们可以在术前进行详细的规划和模拟，确保种植体的位置、角度和深度都达到最优。本书总结了二位作者长期的临床工作经验，详细阐述了数字化种植导板的设计与应用，为读者提供了深入的理解和实用的操作指南。

全瓷材料以其优异的生物相容性和美学性能，成为了现代口腔修复的理想选择。种植体上部全瓷修复有着与天然牙不同的特殊性，本书分牙列缺损种植固定修复和全牙列种植固定修复两部分，从印模制取、CAD设计到CAM加工，详细论述了各步骤的技术要点，展示了如何在实际操作中确保修复体的精度和适配性。

本书还介绍了各类数字化修复材料，详细讨论各自的理化性质与应用特点，只有深入理解材料的本质，才能在临床工作中选择最合适的修复材料。最后的7个精彩纷呈的病例，充分展示了作者团队的精益求精的工作精神，读者可以从中看到数字化导板与全瓷修复的相关技术细节。

本书的一个突出特点是其全面的医技结合。余涛医生和刘海林技师分别从医生和技师的视角，提供了丰富的理论知识和实际操作经验，致力于为读者提供全方位的实践指导。这种医技结合的写作方式，不仅展示了数字化技术在口腔医学中的深度应用，也反映了医生与技师之间紧密合作的重要性。只有通过这种无缝衔接的协作，才能确保每一个治疗步骤的精准和高效，最终实现最佳的治疗效果。

我深信，通过本书的学习，读者能够在实际工作中充分发挥数字化技术的优势，为患者提供更加优质的口腔医疗服务。同时，也希望本书能够激发更多的创新和探索，共同推动口腔医学的发展。

满毅

四川大学华西口腔医院种植科主任、种植教研室主任
中华口腔医学会口腔种植专业委员会副主任委员
全国卫生产业企业管理协会数字化口腔产业分会
副会长
国际骨再生基金中国区执行委员会会长
国际口腔种植学会中国分会候任主席

With a rapid advancing, the introduction of digital technologies has revolutionized the dental medicine and industry, particularly in implant treatment. As a professional in implantology, I am delighted to present the book *Metamorphosis – Clinical and Technological Practices in Digital Surgical Templates and Ceramic Restorations for Implants* by Dr. Yu Tao and Technician Liu Hailin, which offers valuable knowledge and practical guidance for many dentists and technicians.

The success of implant surgery largely depends on the precise placement of the implant, and digital implant guides have emerged to achieve this goal. Detailed planning and simulation before surgery ensure the optimal position, angle, and depth of the implant. This book summarizes the extensive clinical experience of the two authors, elaborating on the design and application of digital implant guides, and providing readers with profound insights and practical operational guidance.

Ceramics have become the ideal material for modern dental restorations due to its excellent biocompatibility and aesthetic qualities. Ceramic restorations on implants possess special characteristics distinct from natural teeth. The book has two chapters of restorations: implant-supported restorations for defected dentitions and implant-supported restorations for the full arch. It details the technical aspects of each step, from impression taking and CAD design to CAM processing, demonstrating how to ensure the accuracy and fit of restorations in practical applications.

Additionally, the book introduces various digital restoration materials, discussing in detail their physicochemical properties and application characteristics. A deep understanding of these materials is essential for selecting the most suitable restoration materials in clinical practice. The final seven exemplary cases fully showcase the author's team's commitment to excellence, allowing readers to appreciate the technical details related to digital guided templates and ceramic restorations.

One prominent feature of this book is its comprehensive integration of clinical and technical knowledge. Dr. Yu Tao and Technician Liu Hailin provided rich theoretical insights and practical operational experience from both the clinical and technical perspectives, offering readers thorough practical guidance. This integrative writing style not only highlights the deep application of digital technology in dentistry but also underscores the importance of close collaboration between dentists and technicians. Only through seamless cooperation can the precision and efficiency of each treatment step be ensured, ultimately achieving the best treatment outcomes.

It's firmly believed that by studying this book, readers will be able to fully leverage the advantages of digital technologies in their work, providing higher quality dental healthcare services to patients. Additionally, I hope this book will inspire further innovation and exploration, collectively advancing the field of dentistry.

Yi Man

Director of Implant Department and Implant Teaching and Research Section, West China Hospital of Stomatology Sichuan University

Vice-Chairman of Chinese Society of Oral Implantology

Vice-President of Chinese Society of Digital Dental Industry

President of National Osteology Group (NOG) China, Osteology Foundation

Chairman-Designate of China Association for International Team for Implantology

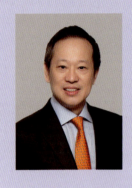

数字化口腔种植技术的全面应用

口腔种植的数字化流程从患者的资料采集开始，贯穿诊断、治疗计划、方案实施等各个环节。数字化口腔种植以终为始，遵循修复导向的治疗原则，相较于传统的种植修复方法，具有更好的预见性、可靠性和安全性。数字化技术全面应用于口腔种植领域，除了赋能给口腔种植医生为患者提供精准的个性化治疗，数字化口腔种植的高准确度，让医生更容易实现微创植牙和即刻负载。

临床实例与技术发展

本书基于临床实例，展示了如何利用数字化导板进行植牙，并实现即刻修复和最终的全瓷修复，整个治疗过程充分体现了医技合作的重要性。我自2003年以来一直关注口腔种植数字化技术的发展，最早接触到的技术是3D打印。当时，要为患者进行数字化导板植牙手术，唯一的途径就是将患者的CT检查的DICOM档案送到比利时的Materialise公司，由他们使用Stereolithography增材制造技术打印颌骨模型和手术导板。虽然所需时间和成本高昂，但这个机会让我开始探索数字化口腔种植的新世界，实在物有所值。现在余涛医生和刘海林先生合著本书，为大家深入探讨已经成熟的数字化口腔种植技术的面貌和精髓。

数字化技术的持续发展

今天，数字化技术持续发展，各种数字化设备不断升级和进步，不仅口腔种植医生掌握的知识和技能不断提高，修复加工方面的发展也日新月异。口腔种植数字化流程的发展已经超过了20年，各种技术从碎片化应用场景到如今的全流程无缝衔接，除了科技的进步，医生团队的协作和加工所技师们的配合与支持也是不可或缺的。余涛医生和刘海林先生这次携手，示范了医技合作的强大力量。

跨学科与跨界别的专业合作

口腔种植是跨学科的专业，数字化口腔种植更是一项跨界别的口腔修复工程。各种数字化影像检查、图像分割技术、影像融合、计算机模拟、3D打印、计算机辅助设计和制造、实时导航、任务自主式种植机器人、人工智能等科技日新月异。只有全身投入、真诚合作，才有机会获得双赢。

余涛和刘海林是年轻一辈中口腔种植专业的佼佼者，生逢其时，正值口腔种植数字化转型的重大机遇中。本书代表了他们在数字化口腔种植方面的合作成果，两人双剑合璧，与广大同行分享他们的经验，教学相长。我在此对两位付出的努力和对行业的热诚表达衷心的赞赏。

周国辉

香港大学牙医学院名誉临床副教授
上海交通大学口腔医学院客座教授
英国皇家外科学院牙科院士
英国皇家外科学院院士

Comprehensive application of digital technology in dental implantology

The digital workflow in dental implantology begins with patient data acquisition and extends through diagnosis, treatment planning, and implementation. Guided by the principles of restorative-driven treatment, digital implantology takes a comprehensive approach, offering improved predictability, reliability, and safety compared to traditional methods.

The widespread adoption of digital technology in implantology empowers dentists to provide precise, personalized treatment. The high accuracy of digital implantology facilitates minimally invasive surgery and immediate loading of implants.

Clinical cases and technological advancements

This book utilizes clinical cases to demonstrate the utilization of surgical guides for implant placement, immediate provisionalisation, and ultimately, full-arch CAD/CAM ceramic restoration. The entire treatment process highlights the importance of collaboration between clinicians and technicians.

My fascination with digital implantology began in 2003 with the advent of 3D printing. Back then, the only way to perform digitally guided implant surgery involved sending the patient's CT scan DICOM files to Materialise in Belgium. They would then use stereolithography to print the jaw model and surgical guide. Despite the high cost and time commitment, this opportunity allowed me to explore the new horizon of digital implantology, making it a worthwhile investment. Now, Doctor Yu Tao and Mr. Liu Hailin have co-authored this book to provide an in-depth exploration of the established landscape and essence of digital implantology.

Continuous evolution of digital technology

Digital technology continues to evolve at a rapid pace, with constant upgrades and advancements in equipment. This progress not only enhances the knowledge and skills of implant dentists but also drives innovation in restorative fabrication. The evolution of digital workflows in implantology has spanned over two decades, transitioning from fragmented applications to seamless integration across the entire process. While technological advancements are crucial, the collaboration within the dental team, including technicians and support staff, is equally vital. Doctor Yu and Mr. Liu exemplify the power of this collaborative approach.

Interdisciplinary and cross-industry collaboration

Implantology is inherently an interdisciplinary field, and digital implantology further amplifies its cross-industry nature. Advancements in digital imaging, image segmentation, image fusion, computer simulation, 3D printing, computer-aided design and manufacturing, real-time navigation, autonomous implant robots, and artificial intelligence continue to reshape the field. Wholehearted dedication and sincere collaboration are paramount to achieving mutually beneficial outcomes.

Doctor Yu and Mr. Liu, both prominent figures in the younger generation of dental professionals, are well-positioned to navigate the transformative era of digital implantology. This book represents the culmination of their collaborative efforts, showcasing their combined expertise and sharing valuable insights with their peers. I commend both authors for their dedication and passion for advancing the field.

James Chow

Honorary Clinical Associate Professor, Faculty of Dentistry, The University of Hong Kong
Honorary Associate Professor, College of Stomatology, Shanghai Jiao-tong University
Fellow in Dental Surgery, Royal College of Surgeons of England
Fellow of the Royal College of Surgeons of England

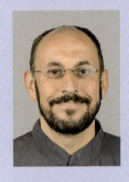

近年来，数字化技术广泛整合于诊断、治疗决策和实施等临床工作，推动了牙科领域的深刻变革。这本名为《蜕变——数字化种植导板与全瓷修复中的医技实践》的书籍探讨了这些进步，聚焦于临床专业知识和尖端技术在数字化手术导板与全瓷修复领域的协同作用。

数字化工作流程与传统牙科实践的融合彻底改变了临床医生诊断、制订计划和执行治疗的方式。这些创新提供了前所未有的精确度、效率和可预测性，提升了医疗质量和对患者的治疗效果。作为牙科专业人员，我们正站在一个新时代的风口，技术和临床智慧的融合正在重塑我们的学科。

通过融合欧洲与中国的优势，我们可以培育更丰富、更多元的牙科领域数字工作模式。这种跨文化合作不仅丰富了科学界，还确保了先进技术对全球更广泛的患者群体的可及性和益处。

数字化手术导板的应用彻底改变了种植学，为种植体植入提供了无与伦比的可靠性。通过详细的病例研究和临床见解，两位作者说明了这些导板如何提高种植修复效果、缩短诊疗时间、提升患者满意度。此外，他们探讨了3D成像和CAD/CAM技术的整合，这些技术已经简化了从规划到执行的整个工作流程。将技术无缝集成到临床实践中，体现了牙科发展的未来方向，精确性和效率并重。

全瓷修复在数字化技术的推动下也受益匪浅。通过数字化设计和制造过程实现的精准性和美学卓越性，为牙齿修复设立了新的标准。本书全面探讨了支撑现代全瓷修复的材料、技能与技术，展示它们在各种临床场景中的应用。利用数字工具定制和完善的修复体不仅改善了治疗结果，还将患者满意度提升至新的高度。

对于我来说，能够表达我对贡献者的感激之情，是一种莫大的荣幸和快乐。正是他们的专业知识和奉献精神，使得本书得以问世。他们的工作体现了推动我们领域进步所必不可少的合作精神。同时，我也要感谢本书的读者们，感谢他们对于专业发展和维护患者健康的热情投入。

在您开始这段数字牙科领域的旅程时，我邀请您考虑这些技术对您的实践产生的深远影响。愿本书成为一座桥梁，为了牙科的未来，连接不同视角，共创美好愿景。

约尔格·纽格鲍尔
美国骨结合学会主席
德国斯泰恩拜斯大学
牙科与口腔医学管理转化研究所数字化牙科教授
德国科隆大学口腔及颅颌面整形外科、
口腔外科和种植科高级讲师

In recent years, the field of dentistry has witnessed a profound transformation, driven by the integration of digital technologies in diagnosis, treatment decision-making, and restorative implementation. This book, *Metamorphosis – Clinical and Technological Practices in Digital Surgical Templates and Ceramic Restorations for Implants*, explores these advancements, focusing on the synergy between clinical expertise and cutting-edge technology in the realm of digital surgical guides and ceramic restorations.

The fusion of digital workflows with traditional dental practices has revolutionized how clinicians approach diagnosis, treatment planning, and execution. These innovations offer unprecedented precision, efficiency, and predictability, enhancing the quality of care and patient outcomes. As dental professionals, we stand at the cusp of a new era where the convergence of technology and clinical acumen is reshaping our discipline.

By drawing on the strengths of both Europe and China, we can cultivate a richer, more diverse understanding of digital workflows in dentistry. This cross-cultural collaboration not only enriches the scientific community but also ensures that advancements are accessible and beneficial to a broader patient population worldwide.

The adoption of digital surgical guides has revolutionized implantology, offering unparalleled reliability in implant placement. Through detailed case studies and clinical insights, the authors illustrate how these guides enhance prosthetic outcomes, reduce chair time, and improve patient satisfaction. Moreover, they explore the integration of 3D imaging and CAD/CAM technologies, which have streamlined the entire workflow from planning to execution. This seamless integration of technology into clinical practice exemplifies the future direction of dental care, where precision and efficiency go hand in hand.

Ceramic restorations have also benefited immensely from digital advancements. The precision and aesthetic excellence achievable through digital design and manufacturing processes have set new standards in restorative dentistry. This book provides a thorough exploration of the materials, techniques, and technologies that underpin modern ceramic restorations, showcasing their application in various clinical scenarios. The ability to customize and perfect restorations with digital tools has not only improved outcomes but also elevated patient satisfaction to new heights.

It is a great honor and pleasure for me to express my gratitude to the contributors, whose expertise and dedication have made this comprehensive book possible. Their work exemplifies the collaborative spirit essential for advancing our field. I also thank the readers of this book for their commitment to professional growth and excellence in patient care.

As you embark on this journey through the landscape of digital dentistry, I invite you to consider the profound impact of these technologies on your practice. May this book serve as a bridge, connecting diverse perspectives and fostering a shared vision for the future of dentistry.

Jörg Neugebauer

President of Academy of Ossteointegration

Professor for Digitization in Dentistry
Steinbeis-University, Transfer-Institute Management of Dental and Oral Medicine, Ludwigshafen, Germany

Senior Lecturer
Department for Oral and Craniomaxillofacial Plastic Surgery
Department for Oral Surgery and Dental Implantology,
University of Cologne, Cologne, Germany

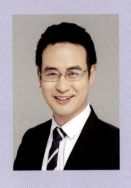

我与刘海林技师认识已久，合作已久。他对口腔种植和修复领域相关技术有非常深刻的理解、有细致入微的钻研，还有孜孜不倦的推广。编写本书的想法，是海林提出的。去年年底，他就与我商讨，随着目前分工细化，除了医生的专业分外科与修复，技师也被分成了手术和修复两类。时常能遇到医生或者技师，外科专业不知修复工作的痛点与难处，修复专业也不理解某些手术其实是不得已才变成增加修复难度的结果。海林便提出，我和他分别是种植外科与修复领域都有涉猎的医生和技师，能否借助数字化种植导板和全瓷修复技术，总结种植手术和种植修复相关临床要点，做一个供读者参考的融合。

数字化种植导板，作为口腔种植手术中的重要辅助工具，凭借其精准的定位和个性化的设计，为口腔种植手术带来了全新的解决方案。数字化种植导板不仅提高了手术的精度和成功率，还减少了手术时间和并发症，为口腔种植患者提供了更加安全、舒适的治疗体验。

虽然种植导板通过数字化技术，降低了对医生经验的依赖，但我也曾经多次在学习班授课时被学员问及导板不准确的相关问题，甚至还有导板辅助下手术之后种植失败的情况。各类临床问题总有各自的复杂之处，本书总结了我与海林合作以来对导板的认识和工作经验，以供读者参考，希望能对各种临床问题的解答提供一些帮助。

全瓷材料在口腔修复领域展现出了其独特的魅力，不仅具有更好的美观性和生物相容性，更能有效降低对牙齿的磨损和刺激，为患者带来更加舒适和自然的口腔修复效果，受到广大患者、医生和技师的青睐。但我们也能看到一些设计不良的种植全瓷修复体，增加了种植治疗的失败风险，如何设计、制作并戴好每一颗种植全瓷修复体，也是值得每一位种植相关医生和技师思考的问题。

我是一位借助数字化技术发展的医生，工作之初，就在数字化技术平台完善的北大口腔门诊部综合科踏上的数字化口腔医学的道路，非常期待能在数字化道路上与诸位读者共同探讨学术，为口腔医学的发展贡献我们的智慧与力量。

著书立言，授业传道，一直是北大口腔门诊部综合科刘峰团队的优秀传统之一。我身在其中，深受熏陶。我十分感谢一路以来每一位医生、护士、技师的支持，还有多位进修生、规培生的协助，让本书最终能成稿问世，让我有机会与广大读者共同传承知识，发展学问，提升技术，不负患者的期待，不负时代的使命！

李涛

2024年5月27日

北京

Dental Technician Hailin Liu and I have known each other and have been collaborating extensively for a long time. He possesses a profound understanding of dental implantation and restoration technologies, demonstrated through meticulous research and tireless promotion. The idea of writing this book was proposed by Hailin. At the end of last year, he discussed with me the current refinement in the division of labor. In addition to the professional division of doctors into surgical and restorative roles, technicians are also categorized similarly. Often, doctors or technicians encounter challenges in restoration work without understanding the surgical specialty, and vice versa. Hailin suggested that, as both doctors and technicians experienced in implant surgery and restoration, we could summarize the essential clinical points of implant surgery and restoration using digital guided templates and all-ceramic restoration technologies to provide a comprehensive guide for readers.

Digital guided templates, as crucial auxiliary tools in oral implant surgery, offer new solutions through precise positioning and personalized design. These templates improve the accuracy and success rate of surgeries, reduce surgical time and complications, and provide patients with a safer and more comfortable treatment experience.

Although digital templates have reduced the reliance on doctors' experience, I have frequently been asked by students about the accuracy of these templates, and there have even been cases of catastrophic failures post-surgery. Clinical problems always have their complexities. This book summarizes my understanding and work experience with these templates since collaborating with Hailin, aiming to help address various clinical issues.

Ceramic materials have demonstrated their unique advantages in oral restoration, offering better aesthetics and biocompatibility, while effectively reducing wear and irritation to the teeth. These materials provide patients with more comfortable and natural restoration effects and are favored by many patients, dentists,

and technicians. However, poorly designed implant-supported all-ceramic restorations can increase the risk of implant treatment failure. Proper design, fabrication, and delivery of each implant-supported all-ceramic restoration is a critical consideration for all implant-related dentists and technicians.

As a doctor who leverages digital technology, I began my career in digital dentistry at the general dentistry department in Clinical Division, Peking University School and Hospital of Stomatology, which has an advanced digital technology platform. I look forward to discussing academic issues with readers and contributing our collective wisdom and strength to the development of dentistry.

Writing books and imparting knowledge has always been a distinguished tradition of our department and Prof. Feng Liu's team. I have been deeply influenced by this tradition. I am immensely grateful for the support of every doctor, nurse, and technician, as well ass the assistance of many advanced students and residents. Their support has enabled the publication of this book, allowing me to share knowledge, develop wisdom, enhance skills together with a wide range of the readers to meet patient expectations and fulfill the mission of our times.

Tao Yu
May 27, 2024
Beijing

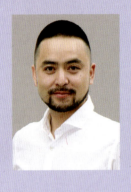

许多年前，当我作为一个刚刚毕业踏入社会的懵懂少年，初涉口腔修复工艺这个行业时，每天在技工室跟在经验丰富的前辈师傅后面，灌石膏、锯代型、制作蜡型、包埋、铸造……烤瓷冠方兴未艾，活动义齿尚属主流，而种植修复作为一个遥远而陌生的概念，还停留在学术会议的专家演讲中。

2012年，欧洲骨结合学会发表的一项共识显示，口腔种植的5年存留率在97.7%，10年存留率在94.9%。"以修复为导向的种植""以生物学为导向的种植"成为越来越多被讨论的话题。数字化技术，尤其是静态导板与动态导航技术的出现，改变了种植外科医生经验主义式的学习曲线，种植手术操作得以向"以终为始"的理想状态逐渐接近。而全瓷修复技术，也由于CAD/CAM和材料学的发展，从事倍功半、难以复制的手工技艺逐步成为事半功倍、易于复制的工业化产品。最终获益的，当然是广大缺牙患者。

然而，在近年来对于数字化种植技术的摸索实践中，我们经历过很多曲折和误区。一些医生，尤其是自由手种植经验相对丰富的外科医生觉得数字化流程烦琐、画蛇添足地增加了就诊次数和时间；一些医生，则认为数字化技术的出现可以让自己一夜之间由新手变为大师，不用花更多的时间积累经验；一些医生把种植导板的制作全盘丢给技师，术中遇到任何困难和偏差，却全归咎于加工厂和技师……

对一项新事物的客观认识，是一个否定之否定的过程。"数字化万能论"和"数字化无用论"都不可取。计算机技术只是给了我们一个精准化种植的工具，但是如何用好这个工具，发挥其优势、规避其短板，需要我们对它的整个实践过程有完整而全面的认知，也需要参与其中的医生、技师、计算机工程师以数字化为载体建立一个扁平化沟通的渠道。

我很庆幸在数字化种植和全瓷修复的实践中遇到了余涛博士。他在北大口腔经过口腔修复学的规范化培训，打下了扎实基础，又在毕业后进入以数字化技术为特色之一的刘峰老师团队持续精进，起点之高令人艳羡，却始终谦逊低调。我们在数字化和全瓷修复领域有着相同的兴趣点，近年来经常一起阅读专业书籍，参加国际顶级专家的课程培训，并且一起完成了很多病例。在合作过程中，我们始终保持着坦诚而无障碍的沟通方式，接近我们认为的最优解。我们相信，通过总结这些病例，并阐述其背后的原理，可以给广大有兴趣从事数字化种植和全瓷修复的医生、技师以实用的帮助，也会鞭策我们不断优化、提升自己，在未来的临床工作中更好地服务广大的患者。

刘海林

2024年5月27日

北京

Many years ago, as a naive young man who had just graduated, I stepped into the field of dental technology as an internship. Every day I followed experienced technicians in the lab, pouring plaster models, making analogs or wax-ups and casting. In China, porcelain crowns were still the most popular products in dental market, and removable dentures were still mainstream ways for rehabilitation. As a distant and unfamiliar concept, implant restoration still remained in expert speeches at academic conferences.

In 2012, a consensus published by the European Association for Osseointegration (EAO) showed that the 5-year survival rate of dental implants was 97.7%, and the 10-year survival rate was 94.9%. "Prosthodontics oriented implant" and "biology oriented implant" have become increasingly discussed topics. The emergence of digital technology, especially static guide and dynamic navigation technology, has changed the empirical learning curve of implant surgeons, and implant surgery has gradually approached the ideal state of "beginning with the end in mind". For ceramic restoration technology, due to the development of CAD/CAM and materials, has gradually evolved from an inefficient manual skill which is difficult to replicate, to an effective industrial product which is reproducible. The ultimate beneficiaries are, of course, the vast majority of patients with missing teeth.

However, in recent years, we have experienced many twists and turns and misunderstandings in the exploration and practice of digital implant technology. Some clinicians, especially surgeons with relatively rich experience in free hand implant surgery, think the digital workflow cumbersome and unnecessary, which increases the number of visits and time of treatment. The other extremes believe that the application of digital technologies can transform themselves from beginners to masters overnight, without spending more time accumulating experience. Some leave the entire work of the implant guide, from design to manufacture, to the technicians. Whatever difficulties or deviations are encountered during the surgeries, the technicians are blamed.

The objective understanding of a new thing is a process of the negation of negation. The theories of "digital omnipotence" and "digital uselessness" are both unacceptable. Computer technology only provides us a precise tool, but how to make good use of this tool, leverage its advantages, and avoid its shortcomings requires us to have a complete and comprehensive understanding of its entire practical process, as well as the dentists, technicians, and computer engineers involved in it to establish a flat communication channel through digital ways.

I am fortunate to have met Dr. Tao Yu in the practice of digital implant treatment and ceramic restoration. He has laid a solid foundation through standardized training in prosthodontics at Peking University School of Stomatology, and after graduation, he joined the team of Professor Liu Feng, characterized by digital technology, to continue to improve. Although his high starting point is admirable, he has always been humble. We share the same interests in the fields of digitalization and all ceramic restoration. In recent years, we have frequently read both classic and pioneering books in digital dentistry, participated in training courses lectured by top international specialists, and completed many cases together. We've been working together with our maximal sincerity and accessibility to approach to the greatest optimum. We believe that by summarizing these cases and explaining their underlying principles, we can provide practical assistance to both dentists and technicians who are interested in digital implant treatment and all ceramic restoration. It will also motivate us to continuously optimize and improve ourselves, and better serve patients in future clinical work.

Hailin Liu

May 27, 2024
Beijing

口腔种植治疗是口腔领域中备受关注的重要内容之一，包括种植手术与种植修复。随着医疗技术的不断发展与临床需求的不断提升，数字化种植导板手术与全瓷种植修复正逐渐成为口腔医学领域的热门研究方向和临床应用焦点。

第1章将阐述数字化导板辅助下种植手术的基本流程与技术要点。本章通过介绍种植导板的临床意义、分类、准确性、局限性等基本认识，以及导板设计、制作过程的技术要点和手术中的操作技巧，希望读者能在临床工作中更好地把握种植导板的使用。

第2章将详细介绍牙列缺损的种植冠、固定桥修复。穿龈轮廓是种植修复体最重要的结构之一，是种植修复比天然牙修复更需要关注之处，本章先深入探讨了种植修复体穿龈轮廓的相关理论与临床实践，然后总结了多种过渡修复体制作方式的技术要点，最后介绍永久修复的物理印模与数字印模两种印模方式及修复体设计、制作和试戴等内容。

第3章将介绍全牙列种植固定修复的基本流程与技术要点。目前用于全牙列种植固定修复的技术方式很多，无法逐一在本书中详细囊括。根据作者团队的工作经验，本章着重介绍一套临床实用性很强的修复流程和相关技术细节。

第4章将介绍氧化锆、玻璃基陶瓷、树脂基陶瓷、聚甲基丙烯酸甲酯等4类用于种植修复的材料，其中以氧化锆这一类种植修复中应用最多的材料为主，分析不同种类氧化锆的特点，总结各自的临床应用。只有深入了解各类材料的性能和特性，才能在临床工作中选择最合适的材料，发挥最大的作用。

第5章展示了作者团队的7个导板辅助下种植手术和全瓷修复的临床病例。这些病例难易不一，从即刻种植到延期种植，从单颗种植到全口种植，有涉及穿龈轮廓的塑形和复制，有不同的即刻过渡义齿制作方式，有辅助准确截骨导板，都涉及了精确的种植体植入。这些病例使用的技术方法，都有非常好的临床实用性。

本书旨在系统性地介绍数字化种植导板和全瓷修复在口腔种植与修复领域的临床应用，我们希望为口腔医生、口腔技师以及相关专业人士提供一份实用的参考资料，为患者谋求更好的临床治疗结果。

Oral implant therapy is a critical area in dentistry, encompassing implant surgery and implant restoration. With the ongoing advancements in medical technology and the rising clinical demand, digital implant guided templates and all-ceramic implant restorations have increasingly become focal points of research and clinical practice in dentistry.

Chapter 1 elaborates on the key aspects of implant surgery and related techniques utilizing digital guided templates. This chapter discusses the clinical significance, classification, accuracy, and limitations of guided templates, along with the design, production process, and operational skills required during surgery. It aims to help readers better understand the use of guided templates in clinical practice.

Chapter 2 provides an in-depth introduction to the restoration of missing teeth using implant crowns and fixed bridges. The emergence profile is a crucial structure in implant restorations, demanding more attention than natural tooth restorations. This chapter explores the relevant theories and clinical practices of the emergence profile in implant restorations, summarizes the technical key points of various interim restorations, and introduces two impression methods for permanent restorations: physical and digital impressions. It covers aspects such as restoration design, fabrication, and delivery.

Chapter 3 presents the basic process and technical key points of full-arch implant-fixed restorations. Given the numerous techniques available for full-arch implant-fixed restorations, this book focuses on a clinically practical restorative process and related technical details, based on the author's team's extensive experience.

Chapter 4 discusses four types of materials used in implant restorations: zirconia, glass ceramics, resin-based ceramics, and polymethyl methacrylate. Zirconia, being the most widely used material, is analyzed in detail, highlighting the characteristics of different types of zirconia and summarizing their clinical applications. A deep understanding of these materials' performance and characteristics is essential to select the most suitable material and maximize its effectiveness in clinical practice.

Chapter 5 presents seven clinical cases of implant surgery and all-ceramic restorations from the authors. These cases range in difficulty, from immediate to delayed implantation, single to full-mouth implantation, involving gingival contour shaping and replication, various methods of immediate transitional prosthesis fabrication, and precise bone cutting guides, all demonstrating accurate implant placement. The technical methods used in these cases have proven to be highly practical in clinical settings.

This book aims to systematically introduce the clinical applications of digital implant templates and all-ceramic restorations in oral implantation and restoration. It seeks to provide a practical reference for dentists, dental technicians, and related professionals, contributing to improved clinical treatment outcomes for patients.

目录　　　　　　　　　　　　　　**CONTENTS**

数字化导板辅助下种植手术的基本流程与技术要点

PROCEDURAL AND TECHNICAL ESSENTIALS OF THE IMPLANT SURGERY ASSISTED BY GUIDED TEMPLATES

第1节　数字化种植导板的基本认识

Section 1 Basics of Guided Templates

数字化种植导板的临床意义

　　如何准确地植入种植体，是每一台种植手术都需要考虑的问题。随着数字化技术在口腔医学中的飞速发展，种植导板（图1）、导航（图2）、机器人（图3）等各类基于患者口腔CBCT、数字印模等三维数据的数字化引导种植技术被用于临床，提高种植体植入准确度，减小手术创伤。其中，数字化种植导板是入门相对容易、应用最广泛的技术，它是指根据患者颌骨解剖结构信息和修复体信息，利用计算机辅助设计与制作技术完成的引导种植窝轴向和/或深度预备以及种植体植入的外科导板。

　　不同病例有着不同的解剖条件，对种植手术的准确度有不同的要求。以下临床场景，对种植手术准确度的潜在要求相对较高。

　　（1）种植位置距离重要解剖结构近。在进行任何手术之前，术者都必须认真评估风险，选择合适尺寸的种植体，设计合理的种植体植入位置、角度、深度，避免损伤下牙槽神经管、上颌窦、邻牙牙根、埋伏牙等重要解剖结构（图4和图5）。

Clinical significance of guided template

In every implant surgery, accurately implanting the implant is a crucial consideration. With the rapid development of digital technology in oral medicine, various digital guided implantation technologies are now available. These technologies are based on patients' oral CBCT and digital impressions, and include guided template (Fig. 1), dynamic navigation (Fig. 2), and robotics (Fig. 3). They are used in clinical practice to enhance the accuracy of implantation and reduce surgical trauma. Among them, guided templates are the most widely used technology with relatively easy entry. Guided templates refer to the guided templates for implant socket axial and/or depth preparation and implant placement completed using computer-aided design and manufacturing technology based on the patient's jawbone anatomy and restoration information.

Different cases have different anatomical conditions, which have different requirements for the accuracy of implant surgery. The following clinical scenarios have relatively higher potential requirements for the accuracy of implant surgery.

(1) The implantation site is close to important anatomical structures. Before any surgery, the operator must carefully assess the risks, choose the appropriate size of the implant, design a reasonable implant position, angle, depth, and avoid damaging important anatomical structures such as the mandibular nerve canal, maxillary sinus, adjacent tooth roots, and impacted teeth (Figs. 4 and 5).

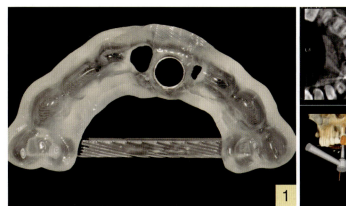

1 数字化种植导板
Guided template

2 导航种植手术系统界面
Dynamic navigation

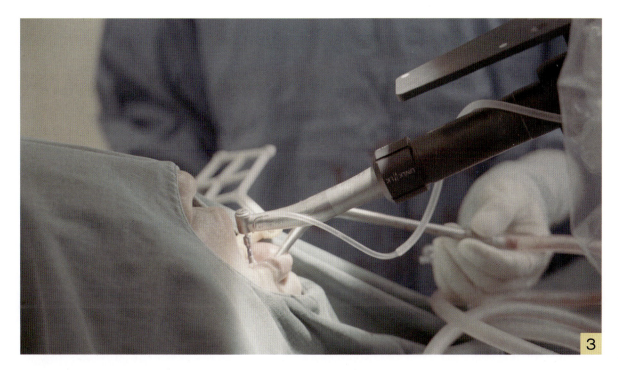

3 种植机器人植入种植体
Robotic surgery

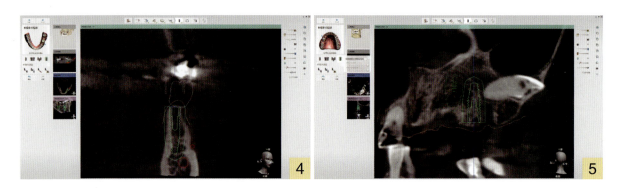

4 种植体距离下牙槽神经近
Close to inferior alveolar nerve

5 种植体距离埋伏牙近
Close to impacted tooth

（2）不翻瓣种植手术。担心手术创伤带来的肿胀与疼痛，是患者害怕甚至拒绝种植治疗的重要原因之一。在合适的条件下，不翻瓣完成种植手术，可以大幅度缩短手术时间，减小手术创伤，降低患者术后痛苦，提高患者对种植治疗的接受程度。但是不翻瓣种植术中术者无法直视牙槽骨形态，会增加损伤重要解剖结构、种植体位置和角度不佳的风险（图6）。

（3）美学区种植。美学区牙槽嵴软硬组织条件有限，错误的种植体轴向、位置可能会带来明显的美学并发症，需要更多的软硬组织增量手术才能弥补，个别情况甚至无法弥补（图7）。

（4）连续多牙缺失需要植入多颗种植体。当连续多牙缺失时，对于最终修复体位置、形态的判断难度增加，种植位点的判断难度也相应增加（图8）。为了降低修复难度，保证修复效果，各种植体之间还需要尽量平行或者处于角度基台对应的角度（图9）。

(2) Flapless implant surgery. Fear of swelling and pain caused by surgical trauma is one of the important reasons why patients are afraid or even refuse implant treatment. In appropriate conditions, performing implant surgery without flaps can significantly reduce the surgical time, decrease surgical trauma, reduce postoperative pain for patients, and improve patients' acceptance of implant treatment. However, in flapless implant surgery, the operator cannot directly visualize the alveolar bone morphology, which increases the risk of damaging important anatomical structures and poor implant positioning and angulation (Fig. 6).

(3) Aesthetic zone implantation. Due to the limited soft and hard tissue conditions in the aesthetic zone alveolar ridge, incorrect implant axis and position may result in significant aesthetic complications, requiring more soft and hard tissue augmentation surgeries to compensate, and in some cases cannot be compensated for (Fig. 7).

(4) When there are multiple missing teeth, multiple dental implants are needed. The difficulty in judging the final restoration position and morphology increases when there are consecutive missing teeth, and the difficulty in determining the implant sites also increases accordingly (Fig. 8). In order to reduce the difficulty of restoration and ensure the restoration effect, it is necessary for the implants to be placed as parallel as possible to each other or at the angle corresponding to the abutment (Fig. 9).

（5）术前制作即刻过渡修复体。为了减少手术当天的治疗时间，术前制作即刻过渡修复体是一种可行的方案。种植体准确植入既定位置，可以直接戴入或者重衬后戴入术前制作的修复体（图10和图11）。

(5) Preoperative immediate transitional restorations are prepared. In order to reduce the treatment time on the day of surgery, preoperative immediate transitional restorations are a feasible solution. The implant is accurately placed in the predetermined position, and the preoperatively fabricated restoration can be directly delivered or delivered after relining (Figs. 10 and 11).

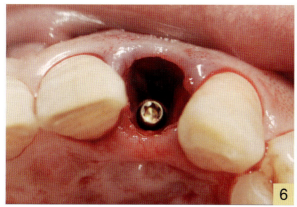

6　不翻瓣种植手术
Flapless implant surgery

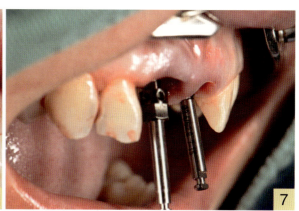

7　美学区种植
Implants in aesthetic zone

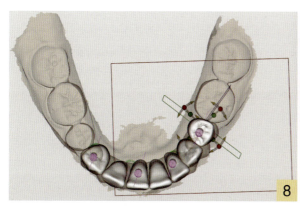

8　连续多牙缺失种植位点设计
Design of continuous multiple implant sites

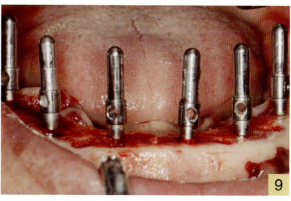

9　连续多颗种植体尽量保持平行
Keeping multiple implants as parallel as possible

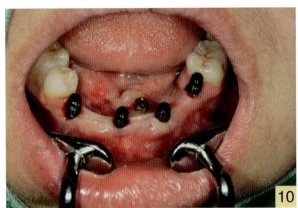

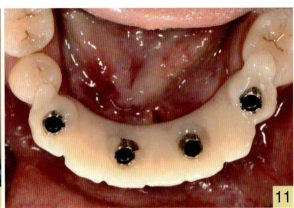

10 准确植入种植体
Accurate placement of the implants

11 重衬术前制作的修复体
Relining the prefabricated restoration

（6）局部骨量有限，常规种植位置和角度骨量不足，但又希望通过种植体位置或者角度的适量改变来避免植骨。比如一些上颌后牙区垂直向骨高度不足但偏腭侧区域又有较多牙槽骨时，如果常规的垂直植入种植体，需要上颌窦底提升，但通过合理范围内的种植体轴向改变，将种植体根尖放在上颌窦腭侧，则可以避免上颌窦底提升（图12）。

以上是临床常见的，对种植准确度有较高要求的情况。但是，并非每次遇到以上情况都必须使用种植导板或者其他数字化种植技术。必须明确，每一个病例都有准确度需求的高低，每位医生都有准确手术能力的强弱，数字化种植技术是提高种植准确度的手段，只有当医生的能力还不足以轻松满足手术需求时，数字化种植技术才能发挥最大的作用。医生可以通过数字化种植技术完成更高难度的病例，但更需要不断提高自身临床水平，不应完全依赖数字化技术。

(6) Bone mass is limited. The bone is not abundant for the normal position and angle of the implant. However, there is a desire to avoid bone grafting by making appropriate changes to the implant position or angle. For example, in cases where the vertical bone height is insufficient in the upper posterior teeth area but there is more alveolar bone in the palatal side area, sinus floor elevation is needed if a conventional vertical implant is used. However, by making appropriate axial changes within a reasonable range and placing the implant apex on the palatal side of the maxillary sinus, the need for sinus floor elevation can be avoided (Fig. 12).

The above are common clinical situations that require high accuracy in implant placement. However, not every situation that meets the above criteria requires the use of guided templates or other digital implant techniques. It must be clear that each case has varying levels of accuracy requirements, each dentist has different levels of surgical accuracy, and digital implant techniques are just means to improve implant accuracy. Only when a physician's ability is not sufficient to easily meet the surgical requirements can digital implant techniques play their maximum role. Dentists can complete more difficult cases with digital implant techniques, but they need to continuously improve their clinical skills and should not rely entirely on digital technology.

数字化种植导板的分类

1. 按引导程度分类

种植导板通过导环将钻针和种植体携带器的运动方向控制在术前设计的种植体轴向上，通过制动装置限制钻针和种植体携带器的运动深度，引导手术步骤准确实施。根据引导程度不同，可以分为先锋钻导板、半程导板、全程导板。

（1）先锋钻导板（图13）。只引导先锋钻的预备，逐级扩孔和种植体植入由自由手完成。先锋钻导板起到很好的定点作用，初步确定种植体植入的轴向与深度，后续自由手逐级备洞和种植体植入还存在一定的变数，是3种导板中受术者经验影响最大的导板。此类导板对手术工具要求最低，只需要先锋钻与导板的导环相适应，其余钻针与自由手手术无异，同一套导环与先锋钻可以用于不同的种植系统。

Classification of guided template

1. Classification by the guiding degree

The guided template controls the movement direction of the drill and implant carrier in the axial direction of the implant designed pre-operatively, and limits the movement depth of the drill and implant carrier with a stop device, guiding the surgical steps to be accurately performed. According to different levels of guidance, it can be divided into pioneer drill guide, half-way guide, and full guide.

(1) Pioneer drill guided template (Fig. 13). The pioneer drilling guided template only guides the preparation of the pioneer drill, while the step-by-step drilling and implantation of the implant are completed by free hand. The pioneer drilling guided template plays a good role in positioning, preliminarily determining the axial direction and depth of implantation. However, the subsequent step-by-step drilling and implantation by free hand still have certain variables. Among the three types of guided templates, this guided template has the greatest impact on the operator's experience. It has the lowest requirements for surgical tools, only needing the pioneer drill to be compatible with the guide sleeve of the guided template. The other drills and free hand operation are no different. The same set of guide sleeves and pioneer drills can be used for different implant systems.

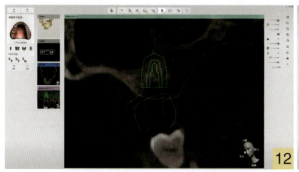

12 适当倾斜以避免植骨
Tilt appropriately to avoid sinus floor lifting

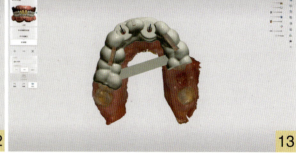

13 先锋钻导板
Pioneer drill guided template

（2）半程导板（图14）。引导先锋钻预备和逐级扩孔，种植体植入由自由手完成。半程导板可以对种植窝洞的位置、轴向、深度都起到良好的引导作用。对于窝洞轴壁密度相对差异较小，种植体植入时侧向力不大的情况，种植体植入的准确性较为有保证；但对于侧向力较大，尤其是即刻种植、早期种植等窝洞一侧有骨、一侧没骨的情况下，种植体植入的准确性一定程度上还依赖于术者的经验。此类导板需要全套专用的钻针，没有控制种植体抗旋结构旋转角度的标记，但使用常规种植体携带器即可，对手术工具的要求高于先锋钻导板。

（3）全程导板（图15）。先锋钻预备、逐级扩孔、种植体植入全程均在引导下完成。全程导板不仅可以完全引导种植体植入既定的位置、轴向、深度，而且可以通过对齐种植体携带器和导环上的特殊标记，控制种植体抗旋结构的角度，即种植体植入时的自转角度，从而实现基台的植入位置也与术前设计保持一致，对于术前制作即刻修复体或者倾斜植入有重要的作用。此类导板需要全套的导板专用钻针和引导型携带器或者引导型种植体，对手术工具的要求最高。

总体而言，排除明显的人为因素之后，引导程度越高，则自由手操作内容就越少，手术准确性就会越高，但这并不意味着所有手术都需要用准确度最高的全程导板。应当充分考虑手术的准确性要求、术者的操作水平、客观现实条件等诸多因素，综合评估后选择导板类型。如果单牙种植，术前已经制作即刻修复体，希望术后马上戴入，则需要控制种植体抗

(2) Half-guided template (Fig. 14). The pioneer drill preparation and step-by-step expansion are guided by the template while the implant is placed by free hand. The half-guided template can provide good guidance on the position, axial alignment, and depth of the implant socket. For cases where the density of the socket walls is relatively consistent and the lateral force when implanting the implant is not large, the accuracy of implantation is relatively guaranteed. However, for cases where the lateral force is large, especially in situations where one side of the socket has bone and the other side does not, such as immediate implantation or early implantation, the accuracy of implant placement still depends to a certain extent on the experience of the operator. This type of template requires a full set of specialized drills, lacks markings to control the rotation angle of the anti-rotation structure of the implant, can be used with a conventional implant carrier, and has higher requirements for surgical instruments than the pioneer drill guided template.

(3) Full-guided template (Fig. 15). The pioneer drill preparation, drilling process, and implant insertion are all done under guidance. The full-guided template not only directs the implant to the intended position, axis, and depth but also controls the implant's anti-rotational structure by aligning special marks on the implant carrier and guide sleeve. This ensures the implant's rotational angle during insertion, guaranteeing the abutment's alignment with the preoperative design. This is crucial for immediate restoration or tilted implantation. Such guided templates require a complete set of dedicated guided template drills and guided carriers or guided implants, with the highest requirements for surgical instruments.

Overall, excluding obvious human factors, the higher the level of guidance, the less manual operation content, and the higher the accuracy of the surgery. However, this does not mean that all surgeries need to be performed with the highest level of accuracy throughout the entire procedure. Factors such as the accuracy requirements of the surgery, the operator's skill level, objective reality conditions, etc., should all be taken into full consideration, and the type of template should be chosen after comprehensive evaluation. If it is a single-tooth

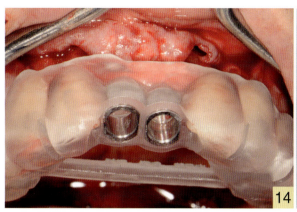

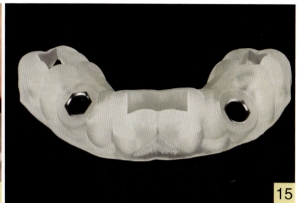

14 半程导板
Half-guide template

15 全程导板（导环与种植体携带器都有六边形结构，二者重叠时种植体抗旋结构旋转角度与术前设计重合）
Full-guided template (both the guide sleeve and the implant carrier have a hexagonal structure, and when they overlap, the rotational angle of the implant anti-rotation structure coincides with the preoperative design)

旋结构的角度，只有全程导板才能满足要求；如果是全口种植，尤其是需要翻瓣去骨的情况，术者也具备一定的自由手种植能力，则先锋钻导板已经能满足大多数情况的需求；如果局部解剖条件较为苛刻，而且术者自身自由手种植能力较弱，一般建议采用全程导板引导手术，以获得最佳的植入效果。

2. 按支持结构分类

（1）牙支持式导板（图16）。此类导板组织面主要与剩余天然牙接触，依靠牙齿提供支持和固位，在连续缺牙数量不多的非游离端牙列缺损、剩余天然牙稳定的情况下应用较多。它的术前准备工作最少，常规口扫和CT就能满足术前数据采集，无需放射导板，部分美学要

implant and an immediate restoration has been prepared before the surgery, with the expectation of wearing it immediately after the surgery, the angle of the implant's anti-rotational structure needs to be controlled, and only a full-guided template can meet the requirements. If it is a full-mouth implant, especially in cases where flap dissection and bone removal are required, and the operator has a certain degree of manual implantation ability, the use of a pioneer drill template can already meet the needs of most situations. If the local anatomy conditions are more stringent, and the operator's own manual implantation ability is weaker, it is generally recommended to use a full-guided template to guide the surgery to achieve the best implantation effect.

2. Classification by support structure

(1) Teeth-supported guided template (Fig. 16). This type of guide mainly contacts with the remaining natural teeth, relying on the teeth to provide support and stability. It is used more frequently in cases of non-free end edentulous dentition with few missing teeth

求高的病例增加相应的照片或者面扫即可；术中不需要固位钉固定导板，但要求术者时刻留意导板的贴合程度与稳定性。

（2）混合支持式导板（图17）。此类导板组织面部分与剩余天然牙接触，部分与缺牙区牙槽黏膜接触，依靠牙齿和黏膜共同提供支持，在黏膜支持部位一般需要固位钉打入牙槽骨进行固位，在游离端缺失牙，或者连续多个跨中线的前牙甚至部分前磨牙缺失情况下应用较多。术前牙列信息采集时，缺牙区牙槽嵴形态十分重要，根据缺牙数量和扫描能力，选择直接制取口内数字印模或者制取物理印模后扫描；术中导板的就位主要依靠牙齿，但更重要的是判断缺牙区导板是否与黏膜完全贴合。

（3）黏膜支持式导板（图18）。此类导板组织面与牙槽黏膜接触，依靠黏膜提供支持，固位钉打入牙槽骨进行固位，在牙列缺失或者余留牙明显松动等牙齿无法提供有效支持的情况下应用较多。术前一般需要制作放射导板，评估未来修复体的美学效果、颌位关系等；术中也常需要借助咬合引导导板的就位，使用固位钉固定导板，甚至可以再次拍摄CBCT确认导板位置与术前设计一致。

and stable remaining natural teeth. Its preoperative preparation is minimal, intraoral digital impression and CT can meet the preoperative data collection requirements, and there is no need for a radiographic guide. For cases with high aesthetic demands, additional photos or face scans may be included. It does not require fixing screws to secure the guide, but the operator should always pay attention to the fit and stability of the guide to ensure proper functioning.

(2) Mixed-supported guided template (Fig. 17). This type of guided template contacts both the remaining natural teeth and the edentulous area mucosa, relies on both teeth and mucosa for support, and generally requires fixation pins to be inserted into the alveolar bone for support in the mucosal support area. It is used more in cases of missing teeth at the free end, or in cases of missing most anterior teeth or even premolar teeth. During preoperative tooth information collection, the morphology of the alveolar ridge in the edentulous area is crucial. Depending on the number of missing teeth and scanning capabilities, either a direct intraoral digital impression or a physical impression followed by scanning can be used. The placement of the guided template during surgery mainly relies on teeth, but more importantly, it is important to determine whether the guided template in the edentulous area fits completely with the mucosa.

(3) Mucosa-supported guided template (Fig. 18). This type of guided template has an organizing surface that contacts the alveolar mucosa for support, with fixation pins inserted into the alveolar bone for stabilization. It is used more often in situations where all teeth are missing in the dental arch, or the remaining teeth are significantly loose and cannot provide effective support. Preoperatively, it is generally necessary to make a radiographic guided to evaluate the aesthetic effect of future restorations, occlusal relationships, etc. During surgery, the use of an occlusal guided template for positioning is often required, with fixation pins securing the guided template in place, and it might even be necessary to re-take a CBCT scan to confirm that the position of the guided template matches the preoperative design.

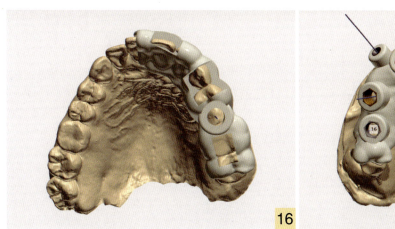

16　牙支持式导板
Tooth-supported guided template

17　混合支持式导板
Mixed-supported guided template

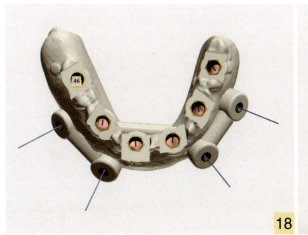

18　黏膜支持式导板
Mucosa-supported guided template

19　骨支持式导板
Bone-supported guided template

（4）骨支持式导板（图19）。此类导板组织面与牙槽骨或颌骨直接接触，依靠骨提供支持。由于CBCT分辨率有限，单纯骨支持的导板较为少见，但在截骨、取骨、骨面开窗等特殊应用中，也有骨支持联合牙支持的联合支持方式。

(4) Bone-supported guided template (Fig. 19). This type of guide relies on direct contact with alveolar bone or jawbone for support. Due to the limited resolution of CBCT, purely bone-supported guides are less common, but in special applications such as osteotomy, bone harvesting, and bone windowing, a combination of bone support and tooth support is also used for joint support.

不同支持类型种植导板对应不同的临床情况，医生并不能像选择引导程度一样选择支持类型。无论何种支持类型的导板，术中导板的就位与稳定是导板下准确手术的前提，是医生需要时刻留意的重要内容。

数字化种植导板的准确性

在种植术后拍摄CBCT，提取种植三维坐标与术前设计比较，评价数字化种植手术准确性，一般有3个指标。植入点偏差：种植体植入点实际位置与设计位置的距离，单位毫米（mm）；根尖偏差：种植体根尖实际位置与设计位置的距离，单位毫米（mm）；植入角度偏差：种植体实际长轴与设计长轴的角度，单位度（°）。

大量的既往研究结果表明，排除明显的人为因素之后，数字化种植导板的平均植入点偏差小于1.5mm，平均根尖偏差小于2mm，平均植入角度偏差小于5°。因此，诸多种植导板设计软件中，植入点安全距离为1.5mm，根尖为2mm。

近两年有不少将导板作为对照组研究导航或者机器人准确性的文章见诸报端，导板的平均植入点偏差约1mm，平均根尖偏差1.5mm，平均植入角度偏差约3°。虽然从研究的结果来看，导板的准确性有提高，但仍不建议随意修改设计软件中的安全距离。

The selection of supporting type is mainly based on the objective clinical situation, rather than the dentist's factor. The placement and stability of the guided template during surgery is the prerequisite for accurate surgery, which doctors need to always pay close attention to.

Accuracy of guided template

After taking CBCT images post-implantation, the extraction of three-dimensional coordinates of implants is compared with preoperative planning to evaluate the accuracy of digital implant surgery. This evaluation is generally based on three indicators: Implantation point deviation, which is the distance between the actual position of the implantation point and the planned position, measured in millimeters (mm); Apex deviation, which is the distance between the actual position of the implant apex and the planned position, measured in millimeters (mm); and Implant angle deviation, which is the angle between the actual long axis of the implant and the planned long axis, measured in degrees (°).

Numerous previous studies have shown that, after excluding obvious human factors, the average deviation of the implantation point of digital guided templates is less than 1.5mm. Additionally, the average root apex deviation is less than 2mm, and the average implantation angle deviation is less than 5°. Therefore, in many guided template design software, the safe distance for implantation points is 1.5mm and for root apex is 2mm.

In the past two years, there have been many articles using guided templates as control groups to study the accuracy of navigation or robotics. The average implant point deviation of the guided templates is about 1mm, the average root apex deviation is 1.5mm, and the average implant angle deviation is about 3°. Although the results of the studies show an improvement in the accuracy of the guided templates, it is still not recommended to change the safety distances in the design software arbitrarily.

另外，我们也看到在部分研究中提到的个案最大根尖偏差甚至能超过5mm，最大植入角度偏差超过10°。因此，充分了解影响导板准确性的因素，避免各类风险，对提高导板手术准确性十分重要。现将影响导板准确性的因素总结如下：

（1）导板种类。多数情况下，同一个临床条件，医生可以选择不同引导程度的导板。导板引导程度越高，准确性越高，即全程导板＞半程导板＞先锋钻导板。CBCT重建的骨面形态受多种因素影响，其准确性并不理想，一般来说，骨支持导板的准确性在不同支持类型的导板里相对较低。其余3种支持类型——牙支持、混合支持、黏膜支持的选择是针对不同的临床条件，比较它们准确性的临床意义并不大。

（2）术前数字印模和CBCT的准确性。数字化种植导板的设计与制作是基于患者的牙列（数字印模）和颌骨（CBCT），这两个数据的不准确，可能使二者无法配准，导板在设计上就是有误差的；也可能影响对术区解剖结构的观察，难以进行合理的种植设计；也可能导致导板组织面设计的不准确，影响导板的就位和稳定。

（3）导板加工的准确性。目前，导板的主流加工方式是3D打印。不同设备、材料、打印条件以及后处理方式可能会影响打印的准确性，打印的准确性直接影响导板完成形态的准确性，影响术中导板的就位与稳定。

In addition, we have also seen that in some studies, the maximum apical deviation of individual cases can exceed 5mm, and the maximum implant angle deviation can exceed 10°. Therefore, understanding the factors that affect the accuracy of the guided template comprehensively, avoiding various risks, is very important for improving the accuracy of the guided template. The factors affecting the accuracy of the guided template are summarized as follows:

(1) Types of guided templates. In most cases, for the same clinical condition, doctors can choose templates with different guidance levels. The higher the guidance level of the template, the higher the accuracy, i.e. full arch template > half arch template > pioneer drill template. The accuracy of bone surface morphology reconstructed by CBCT is influenced by various factors, and its accuracy is not ideal. Generally speaking, the accuracy of bone-supported templates is relatively low among different types of supported templates. The selection of the other three support types (tooth-supported, mixed-supported, mucosa-supported) is aimed at different clinical conditions, and the clinical meaning of comparing their accuracy is not significant.

(2) Accuracy of preoperative digital impressions and CBCT. The design and fabrication of guided templates are based on the patient's dental arch (digital impressions) and jawbone (CBCT). Inaccuracies in these two data sets may result in misalignment of the two, leading to errors in guide design. This misalignment may also impact the observation of anatomical structures in the surgical area, making it difficult to carry out a rational implant design. Additionally, it may lead to inaccuracies in the design of the guide tissue surface, affecting the placement and stability of the guided template.

(3) The accuracy of the guided template processing. Currently, the mainstream processing method of guided templates is 3D printing. Different devices, materials, printing conditions, and post-processing methods may affect the accuracy of the printing, which directly affects the accuracy of the guided templates' completion form and the positioning and stability of the guided templates during the surgery.

（4）导环和导板的就位与稳定。导板通过导环发挥引导作用。导环或者导板产生任何的未完全就位和轻微移动，都无法保证引导钻针或种植体携带器在正确的轴向、位置运动。导板的覆盖范围较大，包含了倒凹区，通常不是整个边缘线都与牙面贴合，这并不利于观察导板的就位情况，需要在贴合的区域开观察窗，便于术中确认导板的就位。导板上的导环能够限制钻针和种植体携带器在既定方向运动，同时也会受到钻针和种植体携带器的反作用力，尤其在从窝洞内退出钻针时，会给导环和导板施加一个脱位力，有时候微小的脱位并不容易被发现。

（5）钻针、手柄或套筒、导环相互之间的间隙（图20）。导环是导板限制钻针运动方向的核心部件。由于半程导板和全程导板都需要用到不同直径的钻针，在导环与钻针之间，通常不同直径的钻针还有一个外径与导环内径匹配、内径与钻针外径匹配的手柄或者套筒，也有部分导板手术工具将在钻针颈部制作粗大的圆柱形结构代替套筒的作用。这些结构之间，必须有一定间隙，才能保证钻针顺利地上下运动。然而过大的间隙又会减弱导板的机械限制作用，降低手术准确性。

(4) The positioning and stability of the guide sleeve and guided template are crucial factors to consider when ensuring the proper functioning of the equipment. Proper alignment and secure attachment of these components are essential for smooth operation and to prevent any potential malfunctions. Regular maintenance and inspection of the guide sleeve and guided template are necessary to address any issues that may arise and to ensure the overall efficiency and safety of the equipment. The guided template guides the drill through the guide sleeve. Any incomplete placement or slight movement of the guide sleeve or guided template cannot ensure the correct axial and positional movement of the guide drill or implant carrier. The coverage area of the guided template is large, including the undercut area. Usually, not the entire edge line is in contact with the tooth surface, which is not conducive to observing the positioning of the guided template. An observation window needs to be opened in the contact area to facilitate intraoperative confirmation of the positioning of the guided template. The guide sleeve on the guided template can restrict the drill and implant carrier in predetermined directions, while also being subjected to counteracts from the drill and implant carrier. Especially when the drill exits the socket, it will exert a dislocation force on the guide sleeve and guided template. Sometimes, a slight dislocation is not easy to detect.

(5) Gaps between drills, handles or drill sheaths, and guide sleeves can lead to inaccuracies in drilling (Fig. 20) . The guide sleeve is the core component that restricts the direction of movement of the drill, ensuring precision and consistency in drilling operations. Due to the different diameters of drills required for both halfway guided templates and full guided templates, there is usually a handle or drill sheath with an outer diameter matching the inner diameter of the guide sleeve and an inner diameter matching the outer diameter of the drill. Some guided template surgical tools will create a thick cylindrical structure at the neck of the drill instead of using a drill sheath. There must be a certain gap between these structures to ensure the smooth up and down movement of the drill. However, excessive gaps will weaken the mechanical limiting effect of the guided template and reduce the accuracy of the surgery.

（6）牙槽骨条件。不均匀的牙槽骨会对钻针和种植体携带器产生侧向力，骨面呈明显斜坡时钻针甚至会打滑，都将降低手术的准确性。另外，也有研究表明，同样类型的种植导板手术，Ⅳ类骨的准确性较Ⅱ类骨和Ⅰ类骨低。

数字化种植导板的局限性

虽然数字化种植导板发展至今，具有较高的种植体植入准确度，一定程度上缩短手术时间，减少手术创伤，但我们依然不能忽视遮挡术区、灵活性低、缺乏手感这3个明显局限性。

导板是通过物理结构直接限制钻针的运动方向，它必须通过导环包裹钻针，多数导板对术区还有明显的覆盖，这种遮挡会降低冷却水对钻针和牙槽骨的降温作用。即使侧方开口的导板，仍然会减弱冷却水的降温作用。术区被遮挡之后，术者无法看到钻针和牙槽骨，如果钻针角度发生偏差，也难以被发现。

(6) Alveolar bone condition. Uneven alveolar bone can generate lateral forces on drills and implant carrier instruments, causing drills to slip on sloped bone surfaces, which will reduce the accuracy of the surgery. Additionally, studies have shown that for the same type of guided template surgery, the accuracy of Class IV bone is lower compared to Class II and Class I bone.

Limitations of guided templates

Although guided templates have developed to a high level of accuracy in implantation, partially reducing the surgery time and minimizing surgical trauma, we still cannot ignore the three obvious limitations: blocking the surgical area, low flexibility, and lack of tactile sensation.

The guided template limits the movement direction of the drill directly through its physical structure. It must be wrapped around the drill by a guide sleeve, and most guided templates also have obvious coverage over the surgical area. This obstruction reduces the cooling effect of the coolant on the drill and the alveolar bone. Even with guided templates that have side openings, the cooling effect of the coolant is still weakened. After the surgical area is covered, the operator cannot see the drill and alveolar bone, making it difficult to detect any deviation in the angle of the drill.

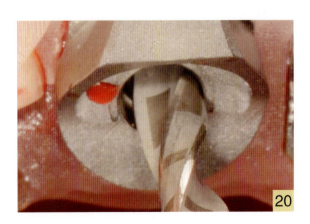

20　钻针与手柄之间的间隙
Gap between reamer and handle

导板是无法在术中进行修改的。一旦导板制作完成，术者只能选择使用或者放弃导板手术，而无法对手术方案进行修改。这要求医生务必在手术前仔细核实和确认手术方案，术中若想修改，只能放弃导板手术。而有时候同一病例可能会有多种种植方案可选择，至少在细节上会有所不同，如果在导板制作完成后，患者提出更改方案设计，就必须放弃导板或者重新制作导板。

在种植备洞的过程中，术者可以明显感受到牙槽骨对种植机的反作用力，针对不同手感的牙槽骨，可以进行备洞策略上的调整，比如阻力大的时候增加钻针提拉次数，依据不同的手感决定是否颈部成型和攻丝钻预备。而导板手术时受导板与钻针之间的作用力影响，医生的手感较弱，完全不同于自由手的情况，备洞策略更多依靠术前读片拟定，术中得到的反馈较少。另一方面，这种手感的缺乏，使得术者不容易总结经验，并不利于手术水平的提高。

The guided template cannot be modified during surgery. Once the guided template is completed, the surgeon can only choose to use or abandon the guided surgery and cannot modify the surgical plan. This requires the doctor to carefully verify and confirm the surgical plan before the surgery. If any modification is desired during the surgery, the guided surgery must be abandoned. Sometimes, there may be multiple implantation options for the same case, at least with some differences in details. If the patient requests a change in the design after the guided template is completed, it is necessary to abandon the template or remake one.

During the process of implantation, the operator can clearly feel the reactive forces of the alveolar bone on the implant machine. For different sensations of the alveolar bone, adjustments can be made in the drilling strategy, such as increasing the number of drill pull-out times when there is high resistance, and determining whether to shape the neck and prepare for threading based on different sensations. During guided surgery, the force between the guided template and the drill affects the surgeon's hand feeling, which is quite different from freehand situations. The drilling strategy relies more on preoperative planning based on radiographs, with less feedback obtained during the operation. On the other hand, this lack of hand feeling makes it difficult for the operator to summarize experiences and is not conducive to improving surgical skills.

第2节　数字化种植导板辅助下手术的基本流程

Section 2 Procedural Essentials of Guided Templates

数字化种植导板的资料采集

1. 数字印模制取

数字印模是以数字化的形式存储和展示患者牙列、牙槽嵴等口腔内部解剖结构形态，可以通过口内数字印模技术直接在患者口内扫描，或者扫描患者的印模或模型。口内数字印模技术的应用比较简便，目前成熟的口内数字印模系统对全牙列扫描的准确度基本能满足种植导板的要求（图21），但由于牙槽黏膜表面光滑，特征点较少，口内数字印模技术直接扫描大范围的黏膜还是有一定的挑战性（图22）。

因此，牙支持式导板可以使用口内数字印模技术直接获得牙列形态；黏膜支持式导板还不能完全使用口内数字印模技术代替物理印模；混合支持式导板如果缺牙间隙不大，黏膜扫描能力较强的口内数字印模系统可以直接获取牙列及牙槽嵴形态，反之，如果缺牙间隙过大，扫描能力不足，则建议制取物理印模后再仓扫印模或者模型。

Data collection for guided templates

1. Digital impression

Digital impression is a digitalized way to store and display the internal anatomical structures of patients' dental arches, alveolar ridges, etc. It can be achieved by directly scanning inside the patient's mouth using intraoral digital impression technology, or scanning the patient's impressions or models. The application of intraoral digital impression technology is relatively simple. Currently, mature intraoral digital impression systems can basically meet the accuracy requirements for full arch scanning for implant guided templates (Fig. 21). However, due to the smooth surface of the alveolar mucosa and fewer characteristic points, direct scanning of a large area of mucosa with intraoral digital impression technology still poses some challenges (Fig. 22).

Therefore, the tooth-supported guided template can directly obtain the tooth arch form using intraoral digital impression technology. However, in case of the mucosa-supported guided template it cannot completely replace physical impressions with intraoral digital impression technology. If the edentulous space of the mixed-supported guided template is not large, an intraoral digital impression system with strong mucosal scanning capabilities can directly obtain the tooth arch and alveolar ridge morphology. Otherwise, if the edentulous space is too large and scanning capabilities are insufficient, it is recommended to take a physical impression first and then scan the impression or model.

口内数字印模技术发展至今，已成为口腔临床最常见的数字化技术之一，在有的医疗机构已经属于患者治疗前的基本检查内容之一，是非常容易获得的临床数据，值得每一位口腔临床医生学习和掌握。虽然在近年来的研究中，各个应用成熟的口内数字印模系统对牙列扫描的准确性都较高，但临床实际应用中，不同系统的扫描速度、流畅度等操作性能还有一定差异。医生需要充分了解口内数字印模系统，选择最合适的系统，掌握必要的操作技巧，才能高效、准确地采集口内数字印模。

（1）定期校准。作为一种精密而复杂的探测系统，口内数字印模系统是需要按要求进行校准的。按照出厂时的要求，定期进行校准，这是口内数字印模系统日常维护的基本内容，否则就会影响所获得数据的准确性。

（2）扫描头灭菌。目前大部分扫描头都可以反复使用，在进入患者口腔时，容易受到唾液、血液污染。扫描头灭菌打包时，可以在内部轻轻塞入洁净的干纱布（图23），以减少高温灭菌对镜片表面的不利影响。反复多次的高温灭菌，有可能会造成扫描头的老化，降低口扫的准确度，建议在安全的次数内使用，以免影响扫描数据的准确性。

（3）避免强光照射患者口腔。在扫描开始之前，应当关闭牙椅灯光、无影灯等高强度的外部光源；对于光照过于强烈的诊室，还应当关闭窗帘，尽量避免杂光干扰。

The development of intraoral digital impression technology has become one of the most common digital technologies in dental clinics. It is already a basic examination before patient treatment in some medical institutions, providing easily accessible clinical data worth learning and mastering by every dental clinician. Although in recent research, various mature intraoral digital impression systems have shown high accuracy in dental arch scanning, there are still certain differences in scanning speed, fluency, and operational performance among different systems in clinical practice. Dentists need to fully understand intraoral digital impression systems, choose the most suitable system, and master the necessary operational skills in order to efficiently and accurately capture intraoral digital impressions.

(1) Regular calibration is essential for the intraoral digital impression system, as it is a precise and complex detection system that needs to be calibrated according to requirements. Following the requirements at the time of manufacture, regular calibration of the intraoral digital impression system is essential for daily maintenance. Otherwise, the accuracy of the data obtained will be affected.

(2) Scan heads sterilization. Currently, most scan heads can be reused, but they are easily contaminated by saliva and blood when entering the patient's oral cavity. When sterilizing and packaging the scan head, clean dry gauze can be gently inserted inside to reduce the adverse effects of high-temperature sterilization on the surface of the lens (Fig. 23). Repeated high-temperature sterilization may cause aging of the scan head, reduce the accuracy of intraoral scanning, and it is recommended to use it within a safe number of times to avoid affecting the accuracy of the scanning data.

(3) Avoid strong light exposure to the patient's oral cavity. Before the scan begins, the dental chair light, shadowless light, and other high-intensity external light sources should be turned off; for rooms with excessively strong light, the curtains should also be closed to minimize the interference of stray light.

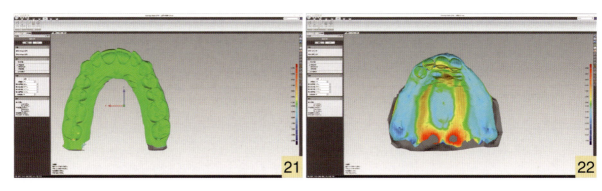

21 全牙列口内数字印模准确性高
High accuracy of intraoral digital impression of teeth

22 黏膜口内数字印模准确性不足
Insufficient accuracy of intraoral digital impression of mucosal

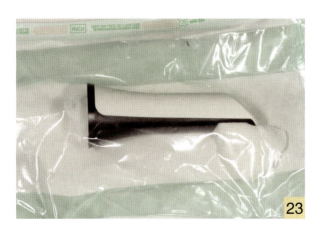

23 扫描头灭菌前塞入干纱布
Insert dry gauze before sterilizing the scanner head

（4）干燥、隔湿。湿润表面会明显影响口内数字印模的制取。在扫描过程中，如果有助手，则能够协助术者牵拉颊、舌黏膜，必要时用强/弱吸管吸走唾液，用三用枪轻吹牙面保持干燥。如果人手不足，使用环形开口器式的橡皮障也起到很好的隔湿效果，牵拉口唇，保持牙面干燥。

(4) Drying and isolation. Liquid surface significantly affects the making of intraoral digital impressions. During the scanning process, the assistant can help the operator retract the cheeks and mucosa of the tongue, use a strong/weak suction device to remove saliva if necessary, and lightly blow the tooth surface with a three-way air syringe to keep it dry. If manpower is insufficient, a good isolation effect can also be achieved by using a rubber dam with a circular opening and retracting the lips to keep the tooth surface dry.

（5）扫描范围。对于牙支持式种植导板，尽量扫描完整牙列，为导板的摆放提供足够的位置。对于混合支持式种植导板，不仅牙列扫描需要完整，缺牙区牙槽嵴也需要扫描完整。对于黏膜支持式导板，如果使用了口内数字印模技术，则建议按照数字化总义齿初印要求，扫描足够的黏膜范围（图24）。

（6）扫描策略。数字印模最大的误差来源是多张三维图像之间的拼接，而不是光学探头本身。建议先流畅、连续完成牙列整体扫描，再补充局部细节；进行第二个面扫描时，建议取景窗内包含部分前一个面的扫描，比如先扫描殆面，再扫描腭侧面时，取景窗内包含部分殆面信息，以提高拼接的准确性（图25）。

2. CBCT拍摄

CBCT的拍摄范围应包括完整的上下颌牙列和上下颌骨。对于CBCT拍摄的运动伪影和金属伪影我们能够尽量去减小。缩短拍摄时间，嘱患者保持静止，可以减少运动伪影；拍摄前，应摘除患者头面部金属饰品、口内含金属成分的可摘义齿、正畸金属托槽；如果固定金属、氧化锆修复体过多，也会产生较多CT伪影，影响种植导板的准确度。而环状伪影、硬化伪影、系统伪影等设备相关的伪影，与设备的维护状态相关。

(5) Scanning range. For teeth-supported implant guided templates, the entire dental arch should be scanned to provide sufficient space for guide placement. For hybrid-supported implant guided templates, not only the dental arch but also the edentulous alveolar ridge areas need to be fully scanned. For mucosa-supported guides, if intraoral digital impression technology is used, it is recommended to scan an adequate mucosal area following the requirements of digital complete denture (Fig. 24).

(6) Scanning strategy. The main reason of error in digital imprinting is the stitching between multiple three-dimensional images, rather than the optical probe itself. It is recommended to first smoothly and continuously complete the overall scan of the dental arch, and then supplement with local details. When performing the second surface scan, it is advisable to include a portion of the previous surface scan within the framing window. For example, when scanning the facial surface after the occlusal surface, include a portion of the occlusal surface information within the framing window to improve the accuracy of stitching (Fig. 25).

2. CBCT

The CBCT scan range should include the complete maxilla and mandible dentition and bones. We can minimize motion artifacts and metal artifacts as much as possible in CBCT scans. Shortening the scan time and instructing the patient to keep still can reduce motion artifacts. Before the scan, the patient should remove any facial metal jewelry, removable dentures with metal components, and orthodontic metal brackets. Excessive fixed metal or zirconia restorations can also cause more CT artifacts, affecting the accuracy of implant guided templates. Ring artifacts, beam hardening artifacts, and system artifacts are equipment-related artifacts that depend on the maintenance status of the device.

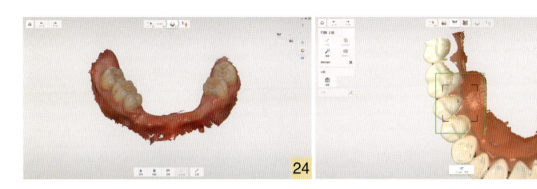

24 黏膜范围足够的数字印模
Digital impression involving sufficient mucosal range

25 扫描腭侧面时包含部分𬌗面信息
Includes partial occlusal surface information when scanning the palatal side

3. 放射导板的制作与应用

当患者全部或者多数牙缺失，无法直接通过剩余牙齿获得稳定、正确的颌位关系时，我们需要放射导板辅助CBCT与黏膜进行数据匹配，辅助医生、技师、患者共同确认后期修复体的形态，从而更好地确定种植体位置和角度，以达到理想的咀嚼功能和美学效果。

制作放射导板的印模要求可参考总义齿要求，部分牙槽嵴低平情况，为了有足够空间放置固位钉，基托边缘可略超过黏膜返折处，但不能干扰放射导板就位并保证咬合状态下放射导板的稳定性。颌位记录和排牙要求都应按照总义齿标准进行，单颌放射导板需要尽量分散放置6～10个放射标志点，锆珠、X线阻射的树脂、牙胶等物质均可以作为放射标志点材料。

3. Preparation and application of radiographic guides

When a patient has lost all or most of their teeth and cannot obtain a stable and correct jaw relationship directly from the remaining teeth, we need to use a radiographic guide to assist in matching CBCT with the mucosa for data alignment. This aids in enabling the doctor, technician, and patient to collectively confirm the morphology of the future restoration, thereby better determining the position and angle of the implant, in order to achieve the ideal chewing function and aesthetic effect.

The production of the template for the radio guided template can refer to the requirements of complete dentures. In cases where the alveolar ridge is low and flat, it's necessary to exceed the edge of the base slightly to the mucosal reflection to have enough space to place the fixing pins. But it must get rid of interfering with the positioning of the radiographic guide and ensuring the stability. Both the jaw relationship record and tooth arrangement requirements should follow the standards of complete dentures. For single-jaw radiographic guide it is preferable to disperse 6-10 radio-opaque marker points as much as possible. Materials such as zirconia beads, X-ray obstructive resin, gutta-percha, etc., can be used as radio-opaque marker materials.

放射导板需要在患者口内试戴，医生、技师、患者三方确认美学效果和颌位关系（图26）。患者佩戴放射导板，拍摄CBCT（图27）。曾经的放射导板还需要进行一次单独的CT扫描，称为双CT扫描。但由于放射导板与人体的X线阻射性质差异很大，需要单独调整CT参数后再进行CT扫描，操作过程较为烦琐。目前更多的处理方式是，使用仓扫或者口扫对放射导板进行光学扫描，获得放射导板的数字印模，包含牙齿排列信息、组织面形态、放射标记点位置。种植设计参考牙齿排列信息，导板组织面形态按照放射导板组织面形态制作，放射标记点可以辅助匹配放射导板形态与CBCT数据（图28）。

数字化种植导板的设计与加工

1. 虚拟修复体的设计

原则上，所有种植设计之前，都应先设计修复体的大致位置与形态。

单颗牙缺失的病例可改变的范围较小，考虑到左右对称、与近远中邻牙协调、与对颌牙咬合关系正常等因素，就能大致设计出修复体形态。当多个前牙缺失，或者多颗前牙需要改变时，应根据美学设计原则，依次确定上颌中切牙中线、上颌中切牙切缘、上颌前牙近远中位置分配、美学区其他牙齿切缘位置、上颌中切牙龈缘、其他牙齿龈缘等变量，最终形成对美学区的整体设计。遇到复杂病例还可以使用面扫、面部照片等数据，辅助美学设计（图29和图30），甚至制作诊断饰面或者诊断义齿，

The radiographic guide should be placed in the patient's mouth for doctors, technicians, and patients to confirm the aesthetic effect and jaw relationship (Fig. 26). The patient will wear the radiographic stent and undergo a CBCT scan (Fig. 27). A separate CT scan, called double CT scan, needs to be done on the previous radiographic stent. However, due to the significant difference in X-ray attenuation properties between the radiographic stent and the human body, the CT parameters need to be adjusted separately before the CT scan, making the operation process more cumbersome. The currently more common approach is to optically scan the radiographic guide to obtain the digital impression, including information on tooth arrangement, tissue surface morphology, and the position of radiographic markers on the guide. The implant design refers to the information on tooth arrangement, the guided template tissue surface morphology is made according to the radiographic guide tissue surface morphology, and the radiographic markers can assist in matching the shape of the radiographic guide with the CBCT data (Fig. 28).

Design and manufacture of guided templates

1. Design of virtual restorations

In principle, the approximate position and form of the restoration should be designed before all implant designs are finalized.

The range that a single missing tooth case can change is relatively small, considering factors such as left-right symmetry, coordination with adjacent teeth in the vicinity, and normal occlusal relationships with opposing teeth, which can design the morphology of the restoration. When multiple anterior teeth are missing, or when multiple anterior teeth need to be altered, variables such as the maxillary central incisor midline, maxillary central incisor incisal edge, maxillary anterior teeth allocation in the proximal, distal, and middle positions, aesthetic zone incisal edges of other teeth, maxillary central incisor gingival margin, and gingival margins of other teeth should be sequentially determined according to aesthetic design principles. This process ultimately forms an overall design for the aesthetic zone. In

确认美学效果和咬合状态。

在使用放射导板的病例中，修复体的形态不仅是有虚拟的设计，而且是制作了实物——放射导板，并在患者口内确认美学效果与颌位关系。设计种植导板时，只需参考放射导板上牙齿形态和排列情况即可。

complex cases, facial scans, facial photos, and other data can be used to assist in aesthetic design (Figs. 29 and 30), and even to create diagnostic veneers or dentures to confirm the aesthetic effects and occlusal status.

In cases where radiographic templates are used, the morphology of the restoration is not only virtually designed, but also physically produced - the radiographic guide, and the aesthetic effect and occlusal relationship are confirmed in the patient's mouth. When designing the implant template, only the tooth form and arrangement on the radiographic guide need to be referenced.

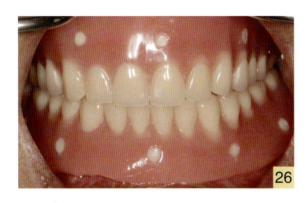

26 试戴放射导板
Wearing of radiographic guide

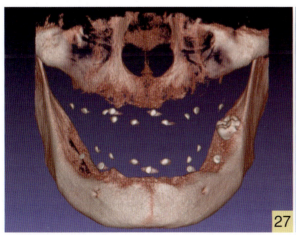

27 戴放射导板拍摄的CBCT
CBCT scan with radiographic guide

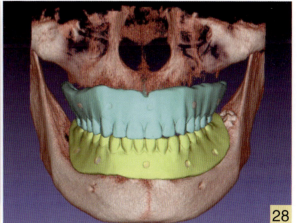

28 配准放射导板数字印模与CBCT
Registration of digital impressions of radiographic guide with CBCT

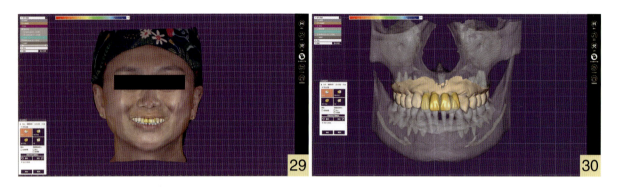

29 面扫辅助下虚拟修复体设计
Design of virtual restoration with facial scanning

30 完成的修复体设计
Completed restoration design

2. 数字印模与CBCT配准

修复体形态和种植导板组织面形态参考的是数字印模，种植体的位置是设计于牙槽骨即CBCT之中。因此，只有数字印模与CBCT配准到一起，才能进行数字化导板的设计。

牙支持式导板和部分混合支持式导板都可以通过分别选取数字印模和CBCT中天然牙的牙尖、点隙等形态分明的结构，将二者配准。使用放射导板的部分混合支持式导板和黏膜支持式导板，依靠放射导板上的多个放射标记点，将数字印模和CBCT配准。

目前，部分设计软件可以自动进行配准，但也可能出现匹配不准确的情况，仍需要手动选择参考点后再进行配准（图31和图32）。

2. Registration of digital impression and CBCT

The morphology of the restoration and template's tissue surface are referenced through the digital impression, while the implant's position is decided by the alveolar bone in CBCT. Therefore, the digital guided template can only be designed when the digital impression is correctly registered with CBCT.

Distinctive structures such as tooth tip, point notch, etc. of natural teeth can be selected in digital impression and CBCT to register tooth-supported templates and some mixed-supported templates. For some other mixed-supported templates and mucosa-supported templates utilizing radiographic guides, the registration of digital impressions and CBCTs depends on multiple radiographic reference points on the radiographic guides.

Currently, some design software can automatically perform registration, but there may be cases of inaccurate matching, which still require manual selection of reference points before registration (Figs. 31 and 32).

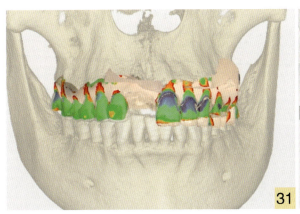

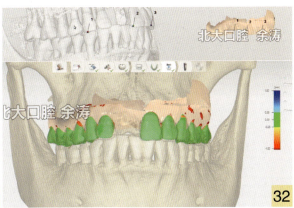

31 发现自动配准数字印模和CBCT不准确
Automatic registration shows inaccuracy

32 手动选择参考点配准数字印模和CBCT
Registration with manual selection of registration points

3. 种植设计

种植设计是数字化种植导板设计中最核心的步骤，是各项种植外科原则的实际体现。以修复为导向，是诸多原则中的一条，可以作为起始点，或者是当作理想状态来考虑。除此之外，更应该关注手术区域局部解剖条件，把种植体放在合适的位置保证外科手术的安全性。另外，还应兼顾患者的年龄、全身状况、对治疗的期望等因素。

前牙区的理想状态是种植体颈部位于最终修复体龈缘下约4mm，种植体周围牙槽骨厚度至少2mm，种植体穿出位置位于修复体舌隆突处（图33）。

3. Implantation design

Implantation design is the most core step in guided template design, which is the practical embodiment of various principles of implant surgery. Restoration-oriented is one of the many principles and can be used as a starting point or considered as an ideal state. In addition, attention should be paid to the local anatomical conditions of the surgical area, placing the implants in the appropriate position to ensure the safety of the surgical procedure. Furthermore, factors such as the patient's age, general condition, and expectations of treatment should all be considered.

In the ideal situation in the anterior region, the implant neck should be positioned approximately 4mm below the final restoration gingival margin, with a minimum bone thickness of 2mm around the implant. The axis of the implant should go through the cingulum of the restoration (Fig. 33).

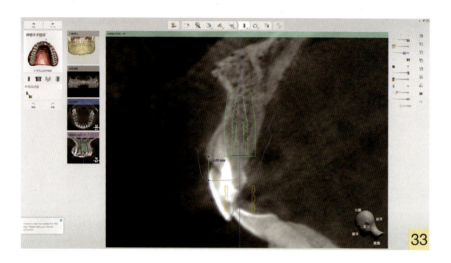

33 理想的种植体位置
Ideal implant position

如果种植体周围牙槽骨厚度不足2mm，可以考虑适当减小种植体颈部直径，单颗上颌切牙使用直径约3.5mm的种植体足矣，部分系统允许下颌切牙植入直径3mm甚至更小的种植体。使用较小种植体唇侧牙槽骨厚度仍不足2mm时，龈缘退缩的风险增加，可以考虑适当的软硬组织增量手术以保持或者恢复牙槽嵴高度及丰满度。在即刻种植病例中，现有唇侧牙槽骨厚度很少能大于2mm，必须保证的是种植体唇侧边缘距离牙槽嵴唇侧边缘的距离大于2mm，最好能在3mm或以上，并且在跳跃间隙内植入低替代率植骨材料，可以有效降低牙龈退缩的风险。如果距离近远中邻牙牙根距离不足2mm时，龈乳头退缩风险增加，尤其是距离不足1.5mm时，龈乳头退缩和邻牙损伤的风险都增加，可以考虑正畸扩大间隙，或者改用其他方式修复。如果是腭侧牙槽嵴顶剩余牙槽骨较薄，腭侧牙龈退缩的风险相对较小，且退缩之后对美学效果影响不大，因此必要时可以

If the thickness of the alveolar bone surrounding the implant is less than 2mm, it should be taken in consideration to appropriately reduce the diameter of the implant neck. A single maxillary central incisor can be restored with an implant diameter of approximately 3.5mm, and some systems allow for implant diameters as small as 3mm or even smaller for mandibular central incisors. When using smaller implants and the buccal bone thickness is still less than 2mm, there is an increased risk of gingival recession. In such cases, consider appropriate soft and hard tissue augmentation surgery to maintain or restore the height and volume of the alveolar ridge. In immediate implant cases, the buccal bone thickness is rarely greater than 2mm, so it is crucial to ensure that the distance between the buccal edge of the implant and the buccal edge of the alveolar ridge is greater than 2mm, preferably 3mm or more. Implanting low-substitution bone materials in the interdental space can effectively reduce the risk of gingival recession. When the distance between the implant and adjacent tooth roots is less than 2mm, the risk of gingival papilla recession increases, especially when it is less than 1.5mm. In such cases of high risks, consider orthodontic expansion of the space or alternative restoration methods. If the remaining alveolar bone on the palatal side is thin, the risk of palatal gingival recession is relatively low, and the aesthetic effect after recession is not significant.

适当将种植体向腭侧移动，以保证唇侧牙槽骨厚度。

前牙种植体理想的种植体穿出位置应位于修复体舌隆突，这样既能保证唇侧软组织足够的空间，腭侧修复体形态不至于过突，还能采用螺丝固位简化修复流程。如果种植体长轴从修复体舌隆突的腭侧穿出，则会使得修复体腭侧过突，可能会影响发音和咬合，增加患者的异物感。如果从切缘穿出，也是较好的轴向，只是修复体需要粘接固位，或者采用角度螺丝。如果从唇面的切1/3穿出，除了固位形式的改变，还可能会减少软组织生长空间，增加唇侧龈缘退缩的风险。以上都是临床可接受的种植体轴向，但我们应尽量避免种植体轴向从修复体唇侧中1/3和颈部1/3穿出。

后牙种植体轴向尽量直立，从修复体𬌗面穿出，正对对颌牙功能尖的非功能尖斜面。如果有倾斜的必要时，也尽量保证穿出位置位于修复体𬌗面；如果受局部解剖条件影响，不得已使用较大角度的倾斜种植，建议以角度基台的角度设计倾斜植入的角度。后牙骨水平种植体应放置在平齐骨面或者骨下0～1mm，软组织水平种植体的光滑颈圈不必植入骨内，仅需要将粗糙面植入骨内即可。对于黏膜很薄的病例，可以适当增加种植体植入深度，以增加未来种植体周围黏膜的厚度。

全口种植固定修复对种植体位置、角度宽容度相对较大，不必要求放在对应的某一个牙位修复体的根方，也不要求种植体之间的完全平行。但应该考虑以下因素：①单颌种植体数量不得少于4颗；②远中悬臂长度＜10mm，尽

In such cases, the implant may be appropriately moved towards the palatal side to ensure adequate buccal bone thickness.

The ideal implant abutment emergence position of the anterior teeth should be located at the cingulum of the restoration, which can ensure a sufficient space for the labial soft tissue, prevent the palatal aspect of the restoration from being over-projected, and simplify the fixation process using screws. If the long axis of the implant emerges from the palatal aspect of the lingual prominence of the restoration, it will cause the palatal aspect of the restoration to be too prominent, potentially affecting speech and occlusion, and increasing the patient's foreign body sensation. If it emerges from the incisal edge, it is also a good axis, but the restoration needs to be cemented or fixed with angled screws. If it emerges from the incisal one-third of labial side, besides the change in fixation form, it may also reduce the space for soft tissue growth, increasing the risk of labial gingival recession. All the above are clinically acceptable implant abutment axes, but we should try to avoid the implant abutment axes emerging from cervical one-third of the restoration.

The axial inclination of the posterior dental implants should be as upright as possible, emerging from the occlusal surface and facing the functional cusp of the antagonist tooth. If there is a need for inclination, it is recommended to ensure that the emergence position is located on the occlusal surface. In cases where greater angulation of the implants is necessary due to local anatomical conditions, it is advised to design the inclined implant at an angle of the angled abutment. Bone-level implants in posterior teeth should be placed at a level bone surface or 0-1mm below the bone surface. The smooth collar of soft tissue-level implants does not need to be placed within the bone; only the rough surface needs to be buried. For cases with thin mucosa, the larger implant depth can be appropriately increased to enhance the mucosal thickness around the implant in the future.

Full-arch implant-supported restorations have relatively large tolerance for implant position and angle. They are not required to be placed directly in line with a specific tooth root, nor do the implants need to be

量增大A–P距离（左右侧近中种植体连线与左右侧远中种植体连线之间的距离）；③种植体之间的连续桥体长度不超过3个牙位（下前牙区除外）；④倾斜种植体角度不大于45°，尽量与角度复合基台角度接近；⑤前牙种植体颈部至切缘距离为12~18mm，如果距离不够，应考虑截骨，加深种植位置，当然截骨还应考虑笑线与义齿–牙龈交接线之间的位置关系；⑥前牙区的螺丝开孔尽量位于舌隆突，后牙区位于𬌗面中央；⑦双侧种植体尽量对称、均匀分布；⑧不侵犯重要解剖结构（上颌窦、鼻腔、切牙管、下牙槽神经管等）；⑨尽量避免植入大量骨缺损处，保证初期稳定性。

总之，种植设计需要考虑诸多因素，数字化导板的种植设计与传统自由手并无本质区别。本书重点在于数字化技术的应用实践，受篇幅限制，仅讲解部分核心的观点，无法详细展开描述种植设计要求，感兴趣的读者可以查阅相关临床参考书。

perfectly parallel. However, the following factors should be considered: ①The number of implants in a single arch should not be less than 4. ②The length of the distal cantilever should be less than 10mm, and the A-P distance (distance between the central implants on the left and right sides and the distal implants on the left and right sides) should be maximized. ③The length of the cantilever bridge between implants should not exceed 3 teeth (excluding the anterior teeth area). ④The angle of tilted implants should not exceed 45 degrees and should ideally be close to the angle of the abutment. ⑤The distance from the neck of the anterior implants to the incisal edge should be approximately 12-18mm. If the distance is insufficient, consideration should be given to bone reduction to deepen the implant position. Of course, bone reduction should also consider the position relationship between the smile line and the denture-gingival junction line. ⑥Screw openings in the anterior area should be located in the lingual prominence, while in the posterior area, they should be in the central fossa. ⑦Implants on both sides should be as symmetrical and evenly distributed as possible. ⑧Avoid encroaching on important anatomical structures (maxillary sinus, nasal cavity, incisive canal, inferior alveolar nerve canal, etc.). ⑨Avoid implanting in areas with significant bone defects as much as possible to ensure initial stability.

In short, planting design needs to consider many factors, and there is no essential difference between digital guided template design and traditional freehand technique. This book focuses on the application of digital technology in practice. Due to space limitations, only some core views are explained, and it is not possible to provide a detailed description of the implantation design requirements. Interested readers can refer to relevant clinical reference books.

4. 导环选择与放置

根据手术工具盒选择对应的导环，一般情况下导环的内径略大于包绕钻针的套筒或者手柄的外径。在不影响就位的前提下，导环的位置应尽量靠近牙槽骨。不翻瓣手术导环不能压迫黏膜，翻瓣手术导环不能压迫牙槽骨（图34和图35）。导环的位置越低，使用的钻针越短，对开口度的要求也越低。后牙种植部分导板工具盒还可以选择侧方开口的导环，使钻针从颊侧进入导环，可用于开口度较小的病例。

设置导环的位置即导环距离种植体颈部的距离时，还应考虑导板手术工具的特殊性，需要与对应的钻针长度相匹配。数字化引导手术需要采用特殊的器械盒，由于导环的内径是固定的，逐级备洞需要的钻针直径并不相同，因此种植导板工具中还包含一套手柄或者套筒，其外侧壁的运动受导环限制，其内侧壁可限制钻针的运动。数字化导板手术的钻针和常规车针并不相同，这是由于考虑了导环的高度、导环到骨面的高度、手柄或者套筒的厚度等，预备车针需要预留出这些长度，才能够获得设计的预备长度。

导环位置（导环底部距离种植体颈部距离）=钻针长度–种植体长度–导环高度–手柄/套筒厚度（图36）。

4. Selection and placement of guided sleeves

When selecting the corresponding guide sleeve for the surgical instrument box, the inner diameter of the guide sleeve is generally slightly larger than the outer diameter of the drill sheath or handle of the drill. The position of the guide sleeve should be as close to the alveolar bone as possible without affecting the placement. For non-flap surgery, the guide sleeve should not compress the mucosa, and for flap surgery, the guide sleeve should not compress the alveolar bone (Figs. 34 and 35). The lower the position of the guide sleeve, the shorter the drill used, and the lower the requirement for the opening width. For the posterior tooth implantation part, a guide sleeve with a lateral opening can also be selected from the guided template toolbox. This allows the drill to enter the guide sleeve from the buccal side, making it suitable for cases with a smaller mouth opening width.

When setting the position of the guide sleeve, the distance between the guide sleeve and the neck of the implant should also consider the specificity of the guided template surgical tools, which need to match the corresponding c length. Digital navigation surgery requires the use of special instrument boxes. Due to the fixed inner diameter of the guide sleeve, the drill diameters required for step-by-step drilling are not the same. Therefore, the guided template tools also include a set of handles or drill sheaths, where the outer wall movement is restricted by the guide sleeve and the inner wall can restrict the movement of the drill. The drills used in guided template surgery are different from the conventional ones. This is because the heights of the guide sleeve, the distance from the guide sleeve to the bone surface, the thickness of the handle or drill sheath, etc., need to be taken into consideration to reserve these lengths for the drill to obtain the designed preoperative length.

The position of the guide sleeve (distance from the bottom of the guide sleeve to the neck of the implant) = length of the drill - length of the implant - height of the guide sleeve - thickness of the handle/drill sheath (Fig. 36).

也有导板工具系统计算的是导环顶部距离种植体的距离，称之为"补偿"，其计算方法也是类似的。补偿=钻针长度–种植体长度–手柄/套筒顶部厚度（图37）。

需要注意的是，如果钻针长度测量时包含了针尖过预备的部分，计算导环位置或者补偿时还需要减去过预备的长度。

The compensation is also calculated by the guide tool system, which measures the distance from the top of the drill sheath to the implant, referred to as "compensation". The calculation method is similar as well. Compensation = length of the drill- length of the implant - thickness of the handle/ drill sheath top (Fig. 37).

When measuring the length of the drill, it is important to subtract any excess length that exceeds the prepared length when calculating the position of the guide sleeve or compensating.

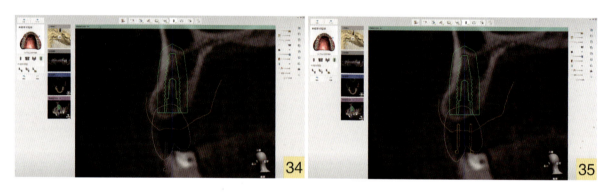

34 不翻瓣手术导环不压迫黏膜
Guide sleeve does not compress mucosa in non-flap surgery

35 翻瓣手术导环不压迫牙槽骨
Guide sleeve does not compress bone in non-flap surgery

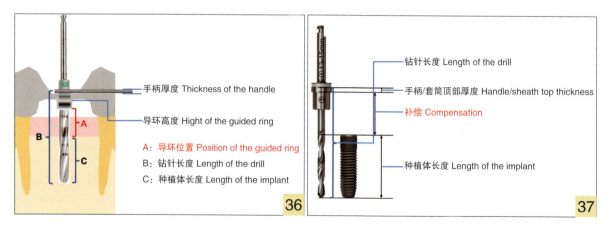

36 导环位置计算示意图
Schematic diagram of guide sleeve position calculation

37 补偿计算示意图
Schematic diagram of compensation calculation

5. 导板边缘线绘制

足够的导板范围可以提供良好的导板稳定性和固位力，导板最好有面式支持，避免仅覆盖后牙线性导板设计。仅单颗后牙种植也建议将导板延伸至对侧牙，至少形成"L"形的导板；前牙种植建议导板至少延伸至前磨牙。导板颊舌面上的边缘线应盖过牙冠的外形高点，但也不应太长影响手术翻瓣，术区可以适当缩小导板覆盖范围便于将冷却水管插入导板下方进行降温（图38）。

6. 观察窗与连接杆的设置

观察窗是在导板合适的位置挖孔，术中通过观察窗确定导板是否完全就位，是否有松动等情况。靠近术区的观察窗还可以减少对术区的遮挡，提供更大的空间，避免手术时干扰种植手机的运动（图39）。观察窗的位置最好位于切缘、牙尖位置（图40），在导板就位后通过这些位置可以直观地看到导板是否与基牙贴合。

连接杆位于双侧导板远中，连接左右两侧导板，使导板形成封闭的环形结构，对减少导板的变形有一定的积极作用（图41）。

5. Drawing the outline line of the guided template

Sufficient template range can provide good template stability and fixation force. It is best to have a surface-supported template to avoid the linear template design that only covers the posterior teeth. For a single posterior tooth implant, it is also recommended to extend the template to the contralateral tooth, at least forming an "L" shaped template. For anterior tooth implants, it is recommended that the template extends at least to the premolars. The edge line on the buccal and lingual sides of the template should cover the outer high point of the tooth crown, but should not be too long to affect the surgical flap. The template coverage range in the surgical area can be appropriately reduced to facilitate the insertion of cooling water pipes under the template for cooling (Fig. 38).

6. Observation window and connecting rod setting

The observation window should be placed in the appropriate position of the guided template. During the surgery, it is used to determine whether the guided template is completely in place, if there is any looseness, etc. Having the observation window near the surgical area can also reduce obstruction, provide a larger space, and avoid interference with the movement of the implant handpiece during surgery (Fig. 39). It is best to place the observation window at the edge of the incisor edge, at the tip of the tooth (Fig. 40), so that after the guided template is in place, it can be visually seen whether the guided template fits with the teeth.

The connecting rod, located in the far middle of the two side fins, connects the left and right sides to form a closed ring structure. This arrangement has a certain positive effect on reducing the deformation of the distal part of the template (Fig. 41).

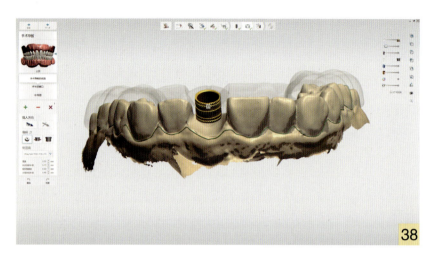

38 导板边缘线绘制
Drawing of the edge line of the guided template

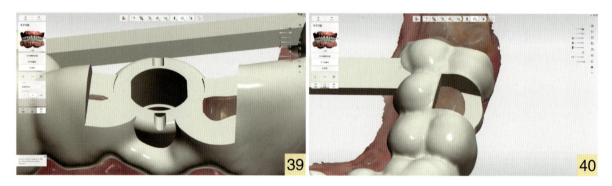

39 术区邻牙上的观察窗
Observation window on the neighboring teeth of the surgical area

40 切缘、牙尖上放置的观察窗
Observation window placed on the cusps of the teeth

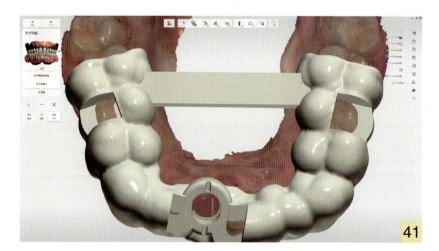

41 连接杆
The connecting rod

7. 3D打印及后处理

3D打印设备和材料的质量固然会影响导板制作的准确度，掌握一些操作细节，也有助于提高导板制作的准确性和效率。安装导环的位置、导板的组织面不能设计支撑（图42）。在方便拆除的前提下，尽量减短支撑杆的长度，有利于缩短打印时间。目前，多数3D打印机都是采用逐层打印的方式进行打印。每层材料之间的堆叠产生的误差，比各层内部的误差较大。因此，在摆放导板时，可以将导环方向垂直于打印平面。

打印完成后，需要从打印平台上取下种植导板（图43），可以用金属铲小心铲断连接导板的支撑杆，并且将支撑杆完全去除。此时的导板可能还未完全固化，还需要二次光照才能完全固化。

8. 导环的粘接

导环是导板上最重要的结构，它必须完全在导板上就位，并且获得良好的固位力，保证手术过程中的稳定。它可以在导板二次固化后，使用树脂水门汀粘接。

数字化种植导板术中要点

数字化导板技术的基本流程并不复杂，主要是在导板完全就位之后，选择适合长度、型号的导板专用车针，按照导板限定的路径，逐级备洞和植入种植体。钻针达到预定的深度时，止动装置发挥作用，钻针不会继续进入过深，整体操作难度不大。

7. 3D printing and post-processing

The quality of 3D printing equipment and materials will indeed affect the accuracy of mold making. Mastering some operational details will also help improve the accuracy and efficiency of mold making. The position to put the guide sleeve and the tissue surface of the template should not be designed with supportive material (Fig. 42). To reduce printing time, try to shorten the length of the supportive rods as much as possible under the premise of easy removal. Currently, most 3D printers use a layer-by-layer printing method. The errors generated by the stacking of materials between layers are larger than the errors within each layer. Therefore, when placing the guided template, the direction of the guide sleeve can be perpendicular to the printing plane.

After printing, the guided template (Fig. 43) needs to be taken off the printing platform. Carefully use a metal shovel to disconnect the support rods from the guide board and completely remove the support rods. At this point, the guide board may not have completely solidified and will require a second exposure to fully cure.

8. Bonding of guided sleeve

The guide sleeve is the most important structure on the guided template. It must be properly positioned on the guided template and obtain good fixation to ensure stability during the surgery. After the secondary curing of the guided template, it can be bonded with composite cementing.

Key points in surgery with guided template

The basic process of surgery with guided template is not complicated. After placing the guided template completely, selecting a guide drill of the appropriate length and type, following the path defined by the guided template, preparing holes step by step, and implanting the implants. When the drill reaches the predetermined depth, the stop mechanism comes into play, preventing the drill from going too deep. Overall, the operation is not very difficult.

1. 手术钻针的选择

种植导板设计完成后，一般会生成钻孔方案，医生可以清楚地看到所需要的工具，一定要求手术开始前就明确所用工具，术中按照清单使用即可。

也有部分导板工具盒里同一直径钻针有多个不同的长度，其长度标识与计划植入的种植体长度对应（图44）。这些钻针的颈部有粗大的圆柱形结构代替套筒的作用，不同长度的钻针该圆柱形结构长度不同，但工作刃长度是一致的（图45）。同一直径备洞时，应从最短的钻针开始预备，逐步更换长钻针至计划植入种植体的长度。因为短钻针的圆柱形结构可以更早地与导环接触，限制钻针的运动方向，而过长的钻针可能在针尖接触骨面时，还未与导环接触，无法限制钻针的运动方向。短钻针在牙槽骨预备出合适的窝洞后，可以引导长钻针的针尖进入窝洞，长钻针继续加深预备时，其圆柱形结构与导环接触，把钻针控制在既定方向上运动。

2. 仔细检查并确认导板就位完全

导板完全就位，才能保证导板所引导的位置、角度正确。导板手术开始之间，必须先试戴导板（图46）。如果发现导板不能完全就位，则必须寻找原因重新制作导板，或者放弃导板手术。每一次下钻和植入种植体之前，也应当核实导板是否完全就位。

1. Selection of surgical drills

After the planting guideboard design is completed, a drilling plan is generally generated, and the surgeon can clearly see the necessary tools. It is essential to clearly define the tools to be used before the surgery begins, and to use them according to the list during the procedure.

In the toolbox, some guide template systems have multiple drills with the same diameter but different lengths, corresponding to the length of the planned implant (Fig. 44). These drills have a large cylindrical structure at the neck instead of a sheath, with different lengths for this cylindrical structure, but the working blade length remains consistent (Fig. 45). When preparing the same diameter holes, start with the shortest drill and gradually change to longer ones until reaching the planned implant length. The cylindrical structure of the short drill can contact the guiding sleeve earlier, limiting the movement direction of the drill. On the contrary, if the drill is too long, it may not contact the guiding sleeve before reaching the bone surface, thus unable to restrict the movement direction of the drill. After preparing a suitable socket in the alveolar bone with the short drill, the tip of the long drill can be guided into the socket. As the long drill continues to deepen the preparation, its cylindrical structure, which contacts the guiding sleeve, controls the movement direction of the drill.

2. Carefully check and confirm that the guided template is securely in place

Before starting the guided template surgery, the guided template must be completely in place to ensure that the position and angle guided by the guided template are correct. It is important to try on the guided template first before proceeding with the surgery (Fig. 46). If the guided template cannot be completely in place, the reason must be found, and the guided template must be remade or the guided template surgery must be abandoned. Before each drilling and implantation of the implants, it should also be verified that the guided template is completely in place.

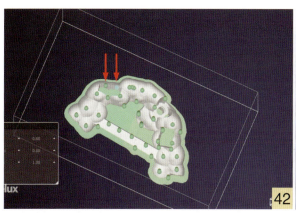

42 去除组织面支撑（红色箭头所指）
Remove the supportive rods on the tissue surface
(indicated by the red arrow)

43 从打印平台取下的导板带有支撑材料
The template removed from the printing platform with
support material

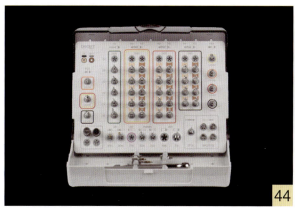

44 以种植体长度标记钻针长度的导板工具盒
Guide box for marking drill length with implant length

45 同一直径不同长度的钻针
Drills of the same diameter with different lengths

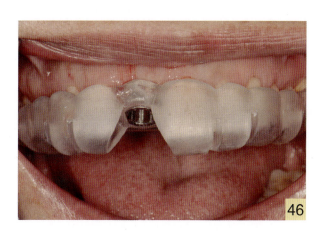

46 术前试戴导板
Preoperative try-in of guided template

导板的边缘可能进入基牙倒凹区，边缘区域未必完全贴合，但是观察窗一般设置在切缘、牙尖等理应贴合的位置，检查导板就位情况时可以检查这些部位的导板是否与基牙完全贴合。

3. 时刻保持导板的稳定状态

试戴导板时，需要评估导板在患者牙列上的稳定性和固位力。如果导板在牙列上非常稳定，不会松动、摇摆，这样的导板可以用于手术；如果在牙列上表现出松松垮垮、容易移动的状态，这样的导板引导的位点和轴向在术中很容易发生移动，出现明显偏差，就不应该在手术中使用，因为其引导的位点和轴向很有可能已出现偏差。

在备洞和种植体植入过程中，术者需要时刻体会导板的稳定性。导板限制钻针的运动方向，钻针也会对导板产生明显的反作用力，引起导板的松动，发生翘动。如果导板固位力良好，术者或者助手用手轻轻按压导板，即可保持导板的稳定；如果导板固位力很差，则非常容易发生松动、移位，术中需要慎重考虑是继续使用导板，还是改为自由手完成手术。

对于混合支持式导板和黏膜支持式导板，应当在不影响备洞和种植体植入的缺牙区牙槽嵴位置，增加固位钉，提高导板的稳定性和固位力。固位钉应尽量分散，呈面式分布。

The edge of the guided template may enter the inverted concave area of the base teeth, and the edge area may not be completely attached. However, the observation window is typically positioned at areas such as the cutting edge and the cusp where attachment should occur. When verifying the positioning of the guided template, you can check if it is fully attached to the base teeth in these specific areas.

3. Always maintain the stability of the rudder

When evaluating the guided template, it is important to assess the stability and retention of the guided template on the patient's dental arch. If the guided template is stable and does not loosen or swing on the dental arch, it can be used for surgery. However, if the guided template is loose and easily moves on the dental arch, it may cause significant deviation during surgery due to shifting of the guiding point and axial direction. In such cases, the guided template should not be used for surgery as it is likely that the guiding point and axial direction have deviated.

During the preparation and implantation process, the surgeon needs to constantly feel the stability of the guided template. The guided template restricts the movement direction of the drill, and the drill also exerts a significant reaction force on the guided template, causing the guided template to loosen and tilt. If the fixation force of the guided template is good, the surgeon or assistant can gently press on the guided template to maintain its stability. If the fixation force of the guided template is poor, it is very easy to loosen and shift; the surgeon needs to carefully consider whether to continue using the guided template or switch to freehand surgery.

For mixed-supportive and mucosa-supported guided templates, additional fixation pins should be added to increase the stability and retention force of the guided template without affecting the alveolar ridge position for osteotomy and implant placement. The fixation screws should be dispersed as much as possible and be distributed in a flat manner.

4. 关于术区降温的考虑

由于导板对术区的遮挡，它必然会影响冷却水的降温作用。导板边缘设计时就应该考虑术中降温的需求，尽量减少导板对术区的覆盖。术中助手可以将冷却水管直接插入导板下方，直冲钻针和牙槽骨，减少导板对降温的不利影响。

钻针转速越快，产热越明显，骨灼伤的风险越高。导板手术中，可以考虑适当降低钻针转速，降低骨灼伤的风险。

虽然导板限制了钻针移动方向，但是术者完全可以控制钻针在轴向上是进入还是退出运动。增加提拉次数，避免一钻到底，可以获得更充分的降温效果，避免升温过快过高。

牙槽骨密度越大，在备洞过程中的产热越多，局部血供越低，则发生骨灼伤的风险越高。比如下前牙区域牙槽骨密度较高，且缺牙间隙往往较小，导板很容易就完全遮挡了术区，此类情况降温效果较差，发生骨灼伤的风险较大，术者必须充分注意备洞手法和冷却水的使用。

4. Considerations about temperature reduction in the surgical area

The presence of the guided template in the surgical area inevitably impacts the cooling efficiency of the cooling water. Therefore, the edge design of the guided template should account for the cooling requirements during the operation and minimize its coverage over the surgical area. The surgical assistant can directly insert the cooling water pipe under the guided template to flush the drill and alveolar bone, thereby mitigating the negative effects of the guided template on cooling.

Higher drill speeds result in increased heat generation and a greater risk of bone burns. During guided template surgery, it may be advisable to reduce the drill speed to lower the risk of bone burns.

Although the guide tube restricts the needle's directional movement, the operator retains full control over the needle's axial entry and exit. By increasing the frequency of withdrawal cycles and avoiding drilling to the maximum depth, a more effective cooling can be achieved, preventing rapid overheating.

Higher alveolar bone density generates more heat during the drilling process, potentially reducing local blood supply and increasing the risk of bone burns. For instance, in the anterior teeth area, where alveolar bone density is higher and interdental spaces are smaller, the guided template often fully covers the surgical area. In such cases, the cooling effect is compromised, and the risk of bone burns is elevated. The operator must pay close attention to drilling techniques and the use of cooling water.

牙列缺损种植修复的基本流程
与技术要点

PROCEDURAL AND TECHNICAL ESSENTIALS OF
IMPLANT-SUPPORTED FIXED RESTORATIONS
FOR PARTIAL EDENTULOUS DENTITIONS

口腔种植的最终目标是制作最佳修复效果的修复体，以帮助患者获得口腔功能和美学的提升。虽然种植治疗是由外科和修复两个专业的治疗手段共同完成的，但两种治疗手段并不是独立分开的两个阶段，各种原则应相互融合，开展外科治疗时应考虑修复相关理念，反之亦然。无论是医生还是技师，从事种植修复工作，自然需要掌握种植修复的相关内容，即使主要从事种植外科工作，也应当了解种植修复相关理念。本章主要介绍牙列缺损种植冠桥修复的穿龈轮廓、过渡修复、永久修复等内容。

The goal of dental implants is to create the best restoration to help patients improve oral function and aesthetics. Although implant treatment is a combination of surgical and restorative approaches, the two treatments are not separate stages, and various principles should be integrated. When performing surgical treatment, considerations should be given to restorative concepts, and vice versa. Both dentists and technicians engaged in implant restorations need to master relevant content. Even if they mainly focus on implant surgery, they should understand restorative concepts related to implants. This chapter mainly introduces the emergence profile, interim restorations, and definitive restorations of dental implants for defected dentition.

第1节　穿龈轮廓

Section 1 Emergence Profile

种植修复体的轮廓，指修复基台从种植体颈部延伸至穿出软组织边缘这部分结构的形态（图1）。轮廓的概念最初并非特别为种植修复体而定，广义上修复体在软组织内的形态均可称为轮廓。

种植体周围软组织明显不同于天然牙的牙周结构。天然牙及其牙周结构中存在穿通纤维，软组织与天然牙表面的结合能力相对较

The concept of the emergence profile refers to the morphology of the structure that extends from the implant neck to the soft tissue margin (Fig. 1). The concept of emergence profile is not originally defined specifically for implant restorations; in a broad sense, the morphology of restorations within the soft tissue can be referred to as the emergence profile.

The soft tissues surrounding implants are markedly different from the periodontal structures of natural teeth. Natural teeth and their periodontal structures have penetrating fibers, providing relatively strong attachment

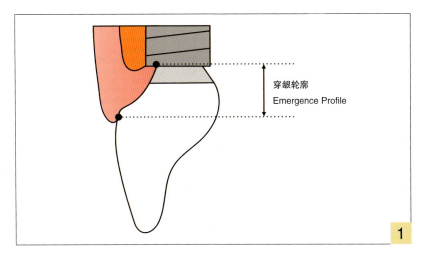

穿龈轮廓
Emergence Profile

1　穿龈轮廓
Emergence profile

强。种植体与周围软组织没有这样的穿通纤维，而是以半桥粒的方式形成较薄弱的结合。因此种植体周围的软组织比天然牙周围软组织更脆弱。

　　另一方面，种植体的植入位置决定上部修复体轮廓的范围比传统修复体更大，种植修复体轮廓的可变化范围更大，对软组织产生的影响也更大。因此，无论是种植过渡修复体，还是永久修复体，其穿龈部分的设计与制作均应遵循一定原则进行，以保证种植体周围软组织的健康与稳定。

前牙区种植修复体的穿龈轮廓

　　种植修复体穿龈轮廓形态可直接改变种植体周围软组织呈现的形态，也能影响种植体周围软组织厚度，前牙区种植修复体的穿龈轮廓需要格外用心设计。

between the soft tissues and the surface of the natural tooth. Implants do not have such penetrating fibers around them; instead, a weaker attachment is formed in hemidesmosome. Therefore, the soft tissues around implants are more fragile than those around natural teeth.

On the other hand, the implantation position of the implant determines that the contour of the above restoration is larger than that of the interim restoration, and the range of variation of the contour of the implant restoration is larger, which also has a greater impact on the soft tissues. Therefore, whether it is an interim implant restoration or a definitive restoration, the design and fabrication of the gingival part should follow certain principles to ensure the health and stability of the soft tissues around the implant.

Emergence profile in anterior region

The emergence profile of the implant restoration can directly change the shape of the surrounding soft tissue of the implant and can also affect the thickness of the soft tissue around the implant. The emergence profile of the implant restoration in the anterior tooth area needs to be carefully designed.

1. 穿龈轮廓大致形态分类

沿种植体长轴作一截面，观察修复体的剖面图，将基台连接种植体的位置与龈缘直线连接，可以用穿龈轮廓与此直线的位置关系，将穿龈轮廓分为3种类型：穿龈轮廓位于该直线内侧（靠近种植体中心轴），称为微凹型；穿龈轮廓位于该直线外侧（远离种植体中心轴），称为微凸型；穿龈轮廓与该直线重合，称为平直型。

（1）微凹型穿龈轮廓（图2）。这种形态的穿龈轮廓的体积较小，对软组织的挤压作用较小，可提供更多的软组织生长空间。大量研究证实，微凹型轮廓有利于获得稳定的种植体周围软组织，减小种植体周围软组织退缩风险。因此，在可能的情况下，种植修复体唇侧应首选微凹型轮廓，以获得更厚的软组织状态，继而更易维持软组织高度和长期的美学效果。

穿龈轮廓并不是越凹越好。过凹的穿龈轮廓可导致修复体对软组织的支撑不足，造成软组织轮廓塌陷，继而造成软组织退缩。过凹的穿龈轮廓意味着修复体厚度的下降，过薄的修复材料不能提供修复体行使功能中所需要的强度。

（2）微凸型穿龈轮廓（图3）。这种形态的穿龈轮廓会挤压软组织的生长空间，降低软组织厚度，可能产生一定的美学风险。对于软组织非常厚但唇侧软组织轮廓仍有丰满度不足的情况，适度增加穿龈轮廓的凸度，甚至呈微凸型，可一定程度向唇侧推移软组织，获得扩增软组织唇侧轮廓丰满度的效果，但一定要谨慎，过凸的穿龈轮廓可能导致牙龈退缩。

1. General types of emergence profile

Cutting along the longitudinal axis of the implant and observing the cross-sectional diagram of the repair site, connect the position where the abutment connects to the implant with the gingival margin. Based on its position relative to this line, the emergence profile can be classified into three types. The emergence profile located inside this line, closer to the center axis of the implant, is called concave type. The emergence profile located outside this line, further away from the center axis of the implant, is called convex type. Lastly, the emergence profile coinciding with this line is called straight type.

(1) Slightly concave emergence profile (Fig. 2). It has a smaller volume, exerts less pressure on soft tissues, and provides more space for soft tissue growth. Numerous studies have confirmed that a concave contour is beneficial for achieving stable soft tissues around implants and reducing the risk of soft tissue recession around implants. Therefore, whenever possible, a concave contour should be preferred on the labial side of implant restorations to achieve a thicker soft tissue status, making it easier to maintain soft tissue height and long-term aesthetic results.

The contour of the gingiva should not be too concave. An excessively concave emergence profile can lead to inadequate support of the soft tissue by the restoration, causing collapse of the soft tissue contour and subsequent recession of the soft tissue. An overly concave emergence profile indicates a decrease in restoration thickness, and a restoration material that is too thin cannot provide the strength needed for the restoration to function properly.

(2) Slightly convex emergence profile (Fig. 3). This type of emergence profile can compress the growth space of soft tissue, reduce the thickness of soft tissue, and may pose certain aesthetic risks. In cases where the soft tissue is very thick, but the labial soft tissue contour is still insufficiently full, moderately increasing the convexity of the emergence profile, even to a slightly convex shape, can shift the soft tissue towards the labial side to some extent. This achieves the effect of enhancing the fullness of the soft tissue labial contour. However, caution is required as excessive convexity of the emergence profile may lead to gingival recession.

若种植体距邻牙间距较大、邻面软硬组织厚度充足，可将邻面的穿龈轮廓设计为微凸型，这样可给修复体间软组织以一定程度的挤压和支撑，有利于塑造和维持龈乳头形态。

必须强调的是，不论是唇侧还是邻面，穿龈变凸均会挤占软组织空间，使其变薄，增加龈缘、龈乳头退缩的风险。因此，穿龈轮廓外凸的设计不是随意而为的，不能形成过凸的状态，否则就有破坏美学效果的可能。

（3）平直型穿龈轮廓（图4）。平直型穿龈轮廓从种植体平台到修复体龈缘的形态大体为直线。这种形态制作简便，介于微凹型与微凸型之间，既为软组织留存一定的空间，同时对软组织保持一定的支撑作用。

修复体舌腭侧可考虑直接形成平直型轮廓。一方面腭侧的美学要求并不高；另一方面平直型修复体的厚度比微凹型更大，可更好地保证修复体强度，同时也没有微凸型对软组织的挤压作用大。

平直型也可以作为微凹型至微凸型的过渡。当软组织塑形时发现需将穿龈轮廓从微凹型向微凸型转换，可先形成平直型轮廓，观察效果。若已达到预期的美学效果，可不必再设计微凸型轮廓。

If the distance between the implant and the adjacent tooth is large and the thickness of the soft and hard tissues on the adjacent side is adequate, the emergence profile on the adjacent side can be designed to be slightly convex. This can provide a certain degree of compression and support to the soft tissue between the restoration units, which is beneficial for shaping and maintaining the gingival papilla morphology.

It must be emphasized that whether it is the labial side or the adjacent side, gingival convexity will occupy soft tissue space, making it thinner, increasing the risk of gingival margin and papilla recession. Therefore, the design of emergence profile should not be done arbitrarily, it should not form an excessively convex state, otherwise there may be a risk of damaging the aesthetic effect.

(3) Flat emergence profile (Fig. 4). It is characterized by a generally straight line from the implant platform to the gingival edge of the restoration. This morphology is relatively easy to create, lying between concave and convex types, providing a certain amount of space for soft tissue retention while also maintaining a certain level of support for the soft tissues.

On the palatal side, the formation of a straight contour can be considered. On one hand, the aesthetic requirements on the palatal side are not high; on the other hand, the thickness of the straight emergence profile is larger than that of the concave type, which can better ensure the strength of the repair body, and at the same time, it does not have the strong pressure effect on soft tissues as the convex type.

The flat profile can also serve as a transition from slightly concave to slightly convex. When shaping soft tissues and transitioning the emergence profile from slightly concave to slightly convex, a flat profile can be formed first for observation of the effect. If the desired visual outcome is achieved, there is no need to create a slightly convex contour.

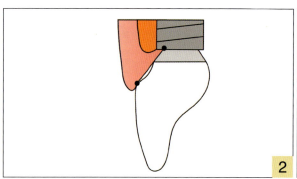

2 微凹型穿龈轮廓
Slightly concave emergence profile

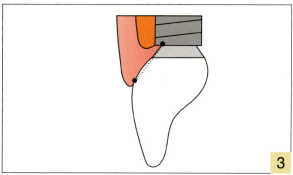

3 微凸型穿龈轮廓
Slightly convex emergence profile

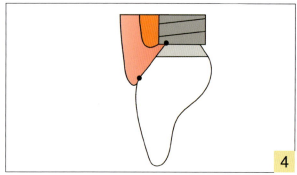

4 平直型穿龈轮廓
Flat emergence profile

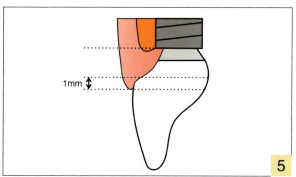

5 关键区域略凸，次关键区域微凹的穿龈轮廓
Slightly convex critical zone, slightly concave subcritical zone

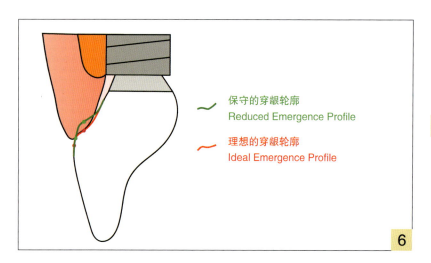

保守的穿龈轮廓
Reduced Emergence Profile

理想的穿龈轮廓
Ideal Emergence Profile

6 龈缘略向冠方移动的穿龈轮廓
Emergence profile slightly moving towards the crown

2. 轮廓的分区

前牙区种植修复美学要求高，修复体形态应根据具体临床情况做出个性化设计和调整，简单的凹与凸并不能完全描述种植修复体的穿龈轮廓，还需要针对不同区域分别处理。

（1）关键区域。这是修复体唇侧龈缘下1mm以内的区域，对龈缘形态的形成和稳定有明显影响，设计和制作需非常准确，应形成与天然牙龈缘下、龈沟内1mm牙体形态类似的略凸形态，以便对龈缘形成良好的支撑，获得必要的形态细节。

（2）次关键区域。这是修复体唇侧龈缘下1mm至种植体平面的区域，相对而言没有关键区域敏感性高，设计和制作时有一定的自由度和灵活度。上述穿龈轮廓大致分出的3种形态实际应用主要是针对次关键区域的形态类型。

所以前牙种植修复体唇侧的轮廓，多数情况是呈现两个曲度的"S"形，关键区域略凸，支撑龈缘；次关键区域微凹，为软组织提供更多生长空间（图5）。如果对软组织管理能力信心不足，种植即刻过渡修复也可以略保守地将龈缘向冠方移动0.5~1mm（图6），为软组织提供更多生长空间，永久修复体时有必要再向根方少量调整即可。

2. Different zones of emergence profile

The aesthetic requirements for implant restoration in the anterior region are high. The shape of the restoration should be personalized and adjusted according to specific clinical conditions. Simple concave and convex shapes cannot fully describe the emergence profile of the implant restoration, and different areas need to be treated separately.

(1) Critical zone. This refers to the region within 1 mm of the gingival margin of the restored tooth, which plays a crucial role in the development and durability of the gingival margin. The design and fabrication need to be very accurate, forming a slightly convex shape similar to the natural teeth margin below the gingival margin and including 1mm of tooth structure within the gingival sulcus. This will provide good support for gingival margin formation and ensure the necessary morphological details are obtained.

(2) Subcritical zone. This is the area from 1 mm below the lip margin of the restoration to the level of the implant platform. In relative terms, the subcritical area is less sensitive, allowing for a certain degree of freedom and flexibility in design and fabrication. The three morphologies identified by the emergence profile described above are mainly intended for the morphology types of the subcritical area.

Therefore, the contour of the anterior implant restoration on the labial side often presents an "S" shaped contour with two curvatures. The critical zone is slightly convex, supporting the gingival margin. The subcritical zone is slightly concave, providing more space for soft tissue growth (Fig. 5). If there is insufficient confidence in soft tissue management, immediate implant interim restorations can conservatively move the gingival margin 0.5-1mm towards the crown (Fig. 6), providing more space for soft tissue growth. A minor adjustment towards the base may be required for the definitive restoration.

后牙区种植修复体的穿龈轮廓

后牙区种植修复对美观要求并不高，需要进行软组织塑形的情况并不多见。但后牙区菌斑控制的难度大于前牙区，种植体周围黏膜炎、种植体周围炎的发病率也高于前牙区。后牙区所承受咬合力量大于前牙区，对修复体厚度有更高的要求。因此后牙区种植修复体的穿龈轮廓以平直型或微凸型为主，便于清洁，厚度足够，且设计简便。

既往研究表明，后牙种植修复体邻面穿龈角度不超过30°，更有利于种植体周围软硬组织的稳定。以下情况均会增加邻面穿龈角度：种植体至邻牙距离变大，种植体深度变小，修复体邻面穿出牙龈的位置向邻牙移动。前两个因素在种植体植入后就已经确定，由此可见外科手术时也必须考虑相应的修复理念。如果在修复时已经是种植体距离邻牙较远、种植位置较浅的情况，也不建议为了减小邻面"黑三角"，将修复体邻面穿出牙龈位置强行向邻牙靠近，最终可能会形成过大的穿龈角度。

临床上如果遇到种植体至邻牙距离合适，深度也合适，但愈合基台直径较小，愈合基台边缘距邻牙较远的情况，也不建议完全按照现有软组织袖口设计一个细小穿龈轮廓，修复体出牙龈后迅速变得粗大，做成"头大脖子细"的形态（图7）。建议更换直径更粗的愈合基台塑形软组织后再修复，或者直接增大穿龈角度制作形态更顺滑的修复体（图8）。后一种方式看似简便，但在戴牙时会有较大软组织阻力，可能需要局麻下少量切开邻面软组织减少

Emergence profile in posterior region

The implant restoration in the posterior region may not require as high aesthetic demands as in the anterior region, and there are fewer cases that require soft tissue sculpting. However, the difficulty of plaque control in the posterior region is greater than in the anterior region, leading to a higher incidence of mucositis and peri-implantitis around implants in the posterior region. The posterior region bears greater occlusal forces than the anterior region, requiring a higher thickness of the restoration. Therefore, the emergence profile of the implant restoration in the posterior region is mainly straight or slightly convex, easy for cleaning, with sufficient thickness and simple design.

Previous studies have shown that the angle of the gingival emergence profile of the distal aspect of posterior implant restorations should not exceed 30°, which is more favorable for the stability of the peri-implant soft and hard tissues. Factors that increase the angle of gingival emergence profile include an increased distance between the implant and the adjacent tooth, a decrease in implant depth, and a movement of the emergence profile towards the adjacent tooth. The first two factors are determined after implant placement, highlighting the need to consider corresponding restorative concepts during surgical procedures. In cases where the implant is far from the adjacent tooth and shallowly positioned, it is not recommended to forcefully move the emergence profile towards the adjacent tooth to reduce the "black triangle", as this may ultimately lead to an excessively large angle of gingival emergence.

In clinical practice, if the distance between the implant and the adjacent tooth is appropriate, and the depth is also appropriate, but the diameter of the healing abutment is small and the edge of the healing abutment is far from the adjacent tooth, it is not recommended to completely design a small emergence profile according to the existing soft tissue cuff design, creating a "big head, small neck" morphology (Fig. 7). It is recommended to replace the healing abutment with a larger diameter to shape the soft tissue before restoring, or to directly increase the emergence profile angle to create a smoother restoration (Fig. 8). The latter method may seem

软组织阻力，甚至个别种植体位置较深的情况可能会有骨阻力，进一步增加戴牙难度。所以医生应参考X线片上种植体与周围牙槽骨关系选择何种方式，同时需要医生具备一定的应变能力。

simpler, but there will be greater soft tissue resistance when wearing the prosthesis, which may require a small incision of the adjacent soft tissue under local anesthesia to reduce the soft tissue resistance. In some cases where the implant is positioned deeper, there may be bone resistance, further increasing the difficulty of wearing the prosthesis. Therefore, doctors should refer to the relationship between the implant and the surrounding alveolar bone on the X-ray to choose the appropriate method, while also needing to have a certain degree of adaptability.

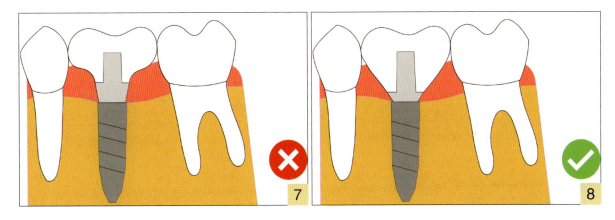

7　"头大脖子细"的修复体
A "large head small neck" restoration

8　穿龈角度增大，形态更顺滑的修复体
A restoration with increased emergence profile angle and smoother shape

第2节 牙列缺损过渡修复

Section 2 Interim Restorations for Partial Edentulous Dentitions

前牙区种植修复对过渡修复的要求较高，因此本节内容主要针对前牙区进行讨论。

种植修复体的负荷时机

国际口腔种植学会将种植体的负荷时机分为：①即刻负荷，种植体植入1周之内；②早期负荷，种植体植入后1周至2个月之间；③常规负荷，种植体植入2~3个月之后。

对于前牙区种植，为获得预期的美学效果，通常建议先戴入过渡修复体进行软组织塑形，待软组织美学效果满意且稳定后，再制作永久修复体。不能进行种植支持过渡修复时，也可采用个性化愈合基台或粘接桥获得类似的效果。前牙区种植过渡修复体有以下几种时机：

（1）种植即刻修复（图9和图10）：即刻种植手术的同时戴入提前设计加工的过渡修复体，或现场设计加工过渡修复体后于种植手术当天戴入。可以即刻修复，但不建议即刻负荷。

The requirements for implant restoration in the anterior region are relatively high, so this section mainly discusses the anterior region.

Timing of loading

The timing of loading on implants is classified as follows: ① Immediate loading, within 1 week after implant placement; ② Early loading, between 1 week and 2 months after implant placement; ③ Delayed loading, 2 to 3 months after implant placement.

To achieve the desired aesthetic effect for anterior area implants, it is usually recommended to first wear an interim restoration to shape the soft tissue. Once the soft tissue aesthetic effect is satisfactory and stable, the definitive restoration can be made. If implant-supported interim restorations cannot be performed, personalized healing abutments or bonded bridges can be used to achieve similar effects. There are several timing options for interim restorations in anterior area implants:

(1) Restoration immediately after implant placement (Figs. 9 and 10): Insertion of a prefabricated interim restoration before immediate implant surgery, or on the same day of implant surgery after on-site design and fabrication of the interim restoration. Immediate restoration is reasonable, but immediate loading is not recommended.

（2）二期手术同期修复（图11）：二期手术中即刻安装过渡修复体，可以即刻负荷。

（3）软硬组织完全愈合后修复（图12）：替换愈合基台的过渡修复体，可以负荷。

(2) Restoration during the second-stage surgery (Fig. 11): It's the restoration inserted during the second-stage surgery, and it can be loaded.

(3) Restoration after complete healing of the soft and hard tissues (Fig. 12): It's the restoration to replace the healing abutment and it can be loaded.

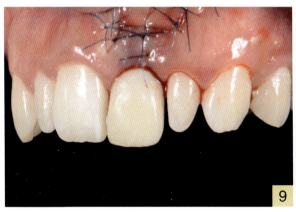

9 即刻种植即刻修复
Immediate implantation and immediate restoration

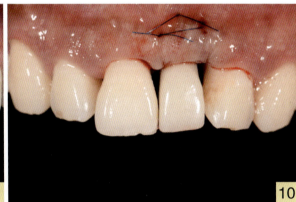

10 延期种植即刻修复
Delayed implantation and immediate restoration

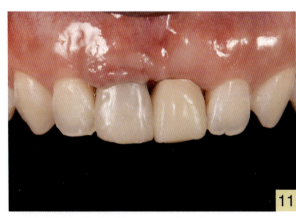

11 二期手术同期修复
Restoration during the second-stage surgery

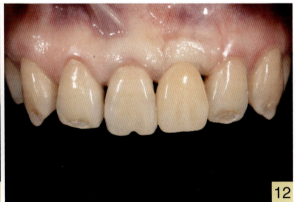

12 软硬组织完全愈合后修复（左上中切牙）
Restoration after complete healing of soft and hard tissues (upper left central incisor)

种植过渡修复体对软组织的作用

1. 保持作用

在安全的前提下，即刻种植同期即刻完成修复体的戴入，可使软组织获得更好的支撑，有机会将术前良好的软硬组织形态维持到修复后，在永久修复前无需调整软组织形态，可大大简化治疗流程。

2. 引导作用

对于早期种植、延期种植或者二期手术同期负荷的患者，由于手术前软组织为牙槽嵴的形态，并非修复体所需要的形态，术后软组织将根据局部实际情况进行愈合。若戴入标准的椎柱形愈合基台，软组织则可被引导成熟为标准的倒锥柱形态，通常与前牙区需要的穿龈袖口形态并不一致；若在这类手术中直接戴入术前设计制作的过渡修复体，或在术中制取印模、设计、加工修复体并即刻戴入，则可引导软组织按照设计好的形态愈合，获得符合美学需求的软组织形态。这个过程称为引导。实现引导作用需要3个重要基础：正确的种植体位点和植入角度，足够的软硬组织量，准确设计和制作的过渡修复体轮廓。

3. 调整作用

对于手术中仅应用愈合基台、未制作过渡修复体的患者，待软组织愈合成熟后，过渡修复体可以将软组织状态调整至理想的美学状态，发挥过渡修复体对软组织的调整作用，也常称为软组织塑形。

Function of the interim restor-ations for the soft tissue

1. Maintaince

Given the safety premises, immediate placement of implants and immediate restoration can provide better support for soft tissues, while also offering the opportunity to maintain the preoperative morphology of soft and hard tissues until final restoration. This simplifies the treatment process significantly before definitive restoration is needed.

2. Guidance

For patients undergoing early or delayed implant placement, or simultaneous loading of a second surgery, the soft tissues before surgery may not be in the ideal form for the alveolar ridge restoration. Postoperative soft tissues will heal based on local conditions. Wearing a standard cylindrical healing abutment can guide soft tissues to mature into a standard inverted cone shape, which may not be suitable for the anterior region. Alternatively, using an interim restoration immediately after the operation can guide soft tissues to heal in a predetermined shape, achieving the desired aesthetic soft tissue morphology. This process is called guided healing. Achieving guidance requires three important fundamentals: correct implant site and insertion angle, sufficient soft and hard tissue volume, and accurately designed and made interim restoration contours.

3. Adjustment

For patients who only use healing abutments during surgery and have not made interim restorations, once the soft tissues are matured, the interim restoration can adjust the soft tissue state to the ideal aesthetic state and play a role in adjusting the soft tissue, also known as soft tissue shaping.

以往进行这种调整、塑形处理时，通常建议采用较柔和的力量进行逐级多次处理。考虑到多次摘戴过渡修复体可能造成软硬组织稳定性下降，有学者建议尽可能减少调整塑形的次数、避免反复摘戴过渡修复体。

过渡修复体的制作要求

1. 良好的稳定性

种植体和过渡修复体就位后均需有足够的稳定性，以免因微动造成边缘骨丧失或骨结合失败。无论是即刻种植还是延期种植的即刻修复，通常建议种植体植入扭矩达到35Ncm时才可进行即刻修复；种植体骨结合完成后种植体的稳定性一般较好，也可以通过测量种植体稳定系数（ISQ）确定种植体稳定后再进行过渡修复。

过渡修复体的中央螺丝扭矩应达到18Ncm，以避免微动（图13）。

2. 咬合接触与邻接触

（1）种植即刻过渡修复。应做到在正中𬌗、前伸𬌗、侧方𬌗等状态下均无咬合接触。为了达到完全无咬合接触的状态，最初的过渡修复体可能较邻牙略短（图14）；可在种植术后3个月、获得骨结合后调整、改善过渡修复体的美学效果。也有学者提出咬合的生理刺激可促进骨结合的理论，但这一理论尚未获得学术界的普遍认可，不能作为临床指导。过渡修复体与邻牙的接触点也应很小范围打开，以避免天然牙的生理动度传递至种植过渡修复体，给

When making such adjustments and shaping processes in the past, it has been generally recommended to use gentle forces for gradual multiple adjustments. Considering that repeatedly wearing and removing interim restorations may cause a decrease in the stability of soft and hard tissues, some scholars suggest minimizing the number of adjustment and shaping times and avoiding repeated removal and wearing of interim restorations.

Fabrication requirements for the interim restorations

1. Good stability

It's critical to the implants and the interim restorations to maintain sufficient stability, preventing marginal bone loss or implant failure due to micro-movement. Whether immediate implantation or delayed implantation with immediate restoration, it is usually recommended that the torque for implant placement reaches 35Ncm before immediate restoration is performed. Implant stability after osseointegration is usually good and can also be assessed through measuring the Implant Stability Quotient (ISQ) before proceeding with interim restorations.

The central screw torque of the transition repair body should reach 18Ncm to avoid micro-movement (Fig. 13).

2. Occlusal contact and proximal contact

(1) Interim restorations immediately after implant placement. It is important to ensure that there is no occlusal contact in the states of central, protrusive, and lateral occlusion. In order to achieve complete elimination of occlusal contact, the initial interim restoration may be slightly shorter than the adjacent teeth (Fig. 14). The aesthetic effect of the interim restoration can be modified 3 months after implantation with achieved osseointegration. Some scholars have proposed the theory that occlusal stimulation can promote osseointegration; however, this theory has not yet been widely accepted by the academic community and cannot be used as clinical guidance. The contact points between the interim restoration and adjacent teeth should also be opened in a small range to avoid

骨结合带来不利影响。

（2）骨结合完成后的过渡修复。此时种植体较为稳定，可以按照永久修复的标准设计咬合接触与邻接触，这样不仅可以调整软组织形态，还可以验证咬合设计是否正确（图15）。

the physiological movements of natural teeth being transmitted to the interim restoration, which may have adverse effects on osseointegration.

(2) Interim restoration after bone integration. At this point, the implant is relatively stable, allowing for the design of occlusal contacts and proximal contacts according to the standards of definitive restoration. This not only allows for adjustment of soft tissue morphology, but also verifies whether the occlusal design is correct (Fig. 15).

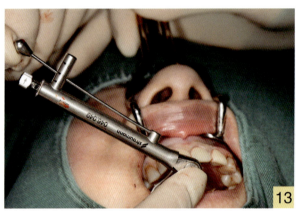

13 旋紧修复基台中央螺丝
Tighten the screw of the restoration

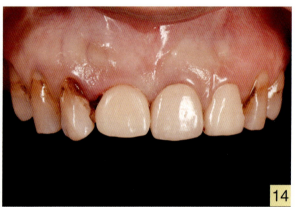

14 种植即刻过渡修复
Interim restorations immediately after implant placemen

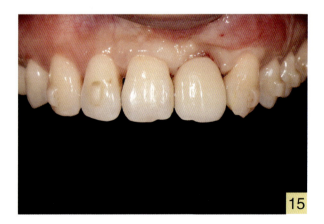

15 骨结合完成后的过渡修复
Interim restoration after osseointegration

3. 固位形式

多数情况下，即使螺丝孔开口在唇侧，也建议采用螺丝固位，可避免粘接性修复体粘接剂溢出、污染手术术区、影响种植体骨结合的问题（图16和图17）。

如果是不翻瓣植入种植体，手术伤口封闭效果非常好，考虑到"one-abutment-one-time"的理念，也可以直接戴入永久修复基台，临时粘接过渡修复体牙冠。

4. 适宜的穿龈轮廓

良好的过渡修复体应能给周围软组织足够的力学支撑，同时给软组织足够的空间生长。过渡修复体的龈缘位置、穿龈轮廓关键区域非常重要，尽量与理想修复体的龈缘一致。

3. Types of fixations

In most cases, even if the screw hole opens on the labial side, it is recommended to use screw fixation, which can avoid issues such as adhesive overflow, contamination of the surgical area, and impact on the osseointegration of the implant (Figs. 16 and 17).

Considering the concept of "one-abutment-one-time", it's also practical to insert the definitive abutment and the temporarily cement interim crown in case of flapless surgery in which the wound can be optimal closed.

4. Appropriate emergence profile

A well-made interim restoration should provide enough mechanical support to the surrounding soft tissues, while allowing enough space for soft tissue growth. The position of the gingival margin and the critical zone of the emergence profile are crucial, and should ideally match those of the ideal restoration.

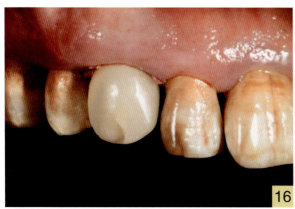

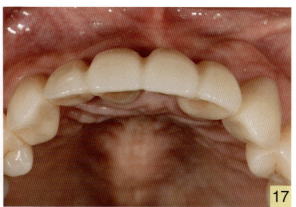

16 唇侧开孔的过渡修复体
Interim restoration of labial side opening

17 舌侧开孔的过渡修复体
Interim restoration of lingual side opening

过渡修复体的制作方法

1. 临时修复基台+术前制作修复体外壳重衬

此方法需要在种植术前制作修复体外壳，用于即刻或者延期种植的即刻修复可缩短手术当天的治疗时间，当然也可以用于其他负荷时机的过渡修复体制作。

修复体外壳形态应与理想修复体形态一致，龈缘务必按照理想龈缘位置或者偏冠方0.5～1mm设计；近远中最好能向邻牙伸出一段小翼，辅助修复体外壳在患者牙列上就位。种植体植入后安装临时修复基台，再将修复体外壳就位，检查修复体外壳与临时基台之间有无干扰，如有干扰，一般建议调磨修复体外壳比较容易。用流动树脂连接修复体外壳与临时基台，确定连接稳定后取下临时基台，继续使用树脂完全连接修复体外壳与临时基台。接下来用树脂堆塑穿龈轮廓，过渡修复体穿龈轮廓的冠方位于修复体外壳的龈缘，根方位于临时基台，因此在龈缘及以下1mm范围内制作略凸的关键区域形态，在更靠根方的次关键区域制作微凹形态。最后修整掉近远中小翼和超出修复体外形的临时基台，打磨抛光，再次消毒，即可到患者口内试戴。

Methods to fabricate the interim restorations

1. Temporary abutment + a shell of the restoration

This method processes as relining a temporary abutment with a shell of the restoration on the implant. It costs less time of surgery and can be utilized in all kinds of timings of loading.

The external shell morphology of the restoration should be consistent with the ideal restoration morphology, and the gingival margin must be designed according to the ideal gingival position or slightly inclined 0.5-1mm towards the crown. It is preferable for the restoration to extend a small wing towards the adjacent teeth in the mesiodistal direction to assist in seating the restoration shell in the patient's dental arch. After implantation of the implant, temporarily mount the restoration abutment, then seat the restoration shell, and check for any interference between the restoration shell and the temporary abutment. If there is interference, it is generally recommended to adjust the restoration shell by grinding. Use flowable resin to connect the restoration shell to the temporary abutment, remove the temporary abutment once the connection is stable, and continue to use resin to completely connect the restoration shell to the temporary abutment. Next, use resin to create the emergence profile, with the transition from the crown contour at the gingival margin of the restoration shell to the root contour at the temporary abutment. Therefore, create a slightly convex key area morphology within 1mm below the gingival margin, and create a slight concavity in the subcritical zone. Finally, trim the small wings and excess temporary abutment that protrudes beyond the restoration shell, polish, disinfect again, and proceed to try in the patient's mouth.

2. 术中制取口内数字印模，CAD/CAM 制作

此方法不必在术前做太多准备工作，可以用于各种负荷时机的过渡修复体制作。口内数字印模系统和扫描杆已是临床常见设备和修复工具，术中制取口内数字印模并不困难。如有椅旁CAD/CAM条件，可以在椅旁直接完成过渡修复体设计与制作；将数据发送至加工厂，加工厂制作后送回临床，这种方式也能实现，但不如椅旁直接CAD/CAM便捷。

术中制取口内数字印模可以采取补扫的方式进行。在手术开始前先制取患者上下颌牙列和咬合的数字印模，将种植位点数据裁剪掉，术中植入种植体后安装扫描杆，仅补扫扫描杆信息即可。术中扫描很难获取软组织形态，而且即使术中获取了软组织形态，也不是理想修复体的软组织形态，设计修复体龈缘时不能参考术中获取的软组织形态。如果术前龈缘位置理想，可以参考术前龈缘；如果龈缘位置需要改变，则需要根据美学原则，设计出修复体的龈缘位置。

此方法制作的过渡修复体穿龈轮廓是与冠部一体化加工而成，穿龈部分表面抛光效果比树脂手工堆塑的方式更好。同时，术中已经获取了种植体位置信息，如果整个过渡期修复体外形没有改动，且不需要改动，可以使用过渡修复体的设计数据，稍作咬合和邻接触等冠方必要的修改，更换材料直接制作永久修复体，不需要重新制取印模，而且同源数据的使用可以保证穿龈轮廓的完美复制。

2. Intraoral digital impression during surgery + CAD/CAM production

This method does not require too much preoperative preparation and can be used for the interim restoration of various loading situations. Intraoral digital impression systems and scan posts are common clinical devices and tools. It is easy to take an intraoral digital impression during surgery. If there are chairside CAD/CAM conditions, interim restoration design and production can be done directly chairside; fabrication in lab and send back to clinic is another solution. This method can also be achieved, but it is not as convenient as chairside way.

During surgery, the intraoral digital impression can be obtained by supplementary scan. Prior to the surgery commencing, impressions of the patient's upper and lower dental arches and occlusion should be taken, ensuring that the data of implant sites are deleted. After implant placement during surgery, the scan post should be installed and only supplementary information should be scanned. It is difficult to accurately obtain the soft tissue morphology during the intraoperative scan, and even if the soft tissue morphology is obtained, it may not accurately represent the ideal soft tissue morphology of the final restoration. Therefore, the soft tissue morphology obtained during surgery should not be used as a reference for designing the gingival margin of the final restoration. If the preoperative gingival margin position is ideal, it can be used as a reference; if the gingival margin position needs to be changed, the gingival margin position of the restoration should be designed according to aesthetic principles.

The interim restoration made by this method integrates with the contour of the coronal portion. The polished surface of the transgingival portion is better than the resin manual shaping method. During the surgery, the implant position information has been obtained. If the overall shape of the interim restoration remains unchanged and no modifications are needed, the design data of the interim restoration can be used. With slight adjustments to the occlusion and crown-to-crown contacts, a definitive restoration can be directly fabricated without the need to take a new impression. The use of homologous data may contribute to achieving a more accurate replication of the emergence profile.

3. 术前完全预成过渡修复体

导板设计完成后能导出包含种植设计的牙列数据，术前可以在此虚拟设计的种植体上设计并制作过渡修复体。全程导板引导下植入种植体，种植体的位置、轴向、抗旋结构角度误差较小，对于单牙种植修复，是能够实现戴入术前制作的过渡修复体，大幅缩短手术和即刻修复的总时间（图18～图21）。

3. Preoperative fully prefabricated interim restoration

After the guide plate design is completed, it can export the tooth row data containing the planting design. Before the procedure, interim restoration can be designed and applied to the virtual implant that has been designed on this implant. The implant is placed under the guidance of the template throughout the process. The position, axial direction, and anti-rotation structural angle error of the implant are small. For single-tooth implant restorations, it is possible to achieve the interim restoration made before the operation, greatly shortening the total time of surgery and immediate restoration (Figs. 18 to 21).

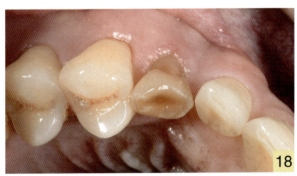

18 13种植治疗前
Tooth 13 before treatment

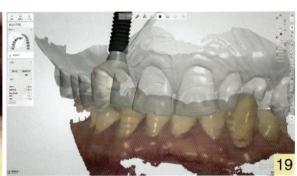

19 过渡修复体设计
Interim restoration design

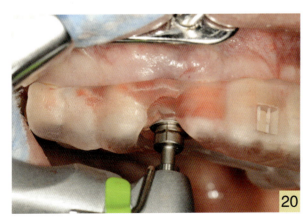
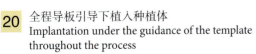

20 全程导板引导下植入种植体
Implantation under the guidance of the template throughout the process

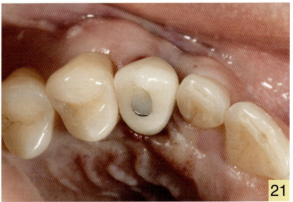

21 即刻戴入过渡修复体
Immediate insertion of the interim restoration

4. 其他制作方法

临时修复体基台上还可以完全使用树脂堆塑过渡修复体形态，或者使用拔除的患牙进行重衬并制作过渡修复体。但前者对医生的操作能力要求较高，尤其是唇面形态的制作和龈缘的确定；后者需要一颗形态完好，尤其是颈部完整的牙冠，除根折和自腭侧至唇侧的冠根折以外，临床上很少遇到此类牙冠完整的患牙拔除后还满足即刻种植的适应证。

术中使用转移杆和流动树脂制取局部印模，转技工室制作过渡修复体，也曾是较常见的方式。但随着数字化技术的发展，制取种植修复的口内数字印模已非常普遍，且用在术中污染术区的风险更小。因此，如果需要术中制取印模，则明确建议使用口内数字印模。

4. Other production methods

Temporary restoration can completely be made on the abutment with resin, or by using the extracted tooth for re-lining and making the interim restoration. The former option requires higher operating capabilities for dentists, especially in the fabrication of lip morphology and determination of gingival margins. The latter option requires a tooth with intact morphology, specifically a crown with a complete neck. Situations where a complete crown tooth can be extracted and immediately meet the indications for immediate implantation are rarely encountered in clinical practice.

It used to be classical to take partial impression during surgery and fabricate the interim restoration in lab. However, with the development of digital technology, intraoral digital impressions for implant restorations have become very common, resulting in a lower risk of contaminating the surgical site during the procedure. Therefore, if intraoperative impressions are needed, it is strongly recommended to use digital intraoral impressions.

第3节　牙列缺损永久修复

Section 3 Definitive Restorations for Partial Edentulous Dentitions

物理印模

种植冠桥修复一般制取种植体水平的印模，是为了将口内种植体位置信息准确转移到口外模型中，需要转移杆连接种植体并固定在印模内，取出口外后再连接种植体替代体，灌制石膏模型。

1. 单颗后牙

种植修复转移杆有开窗式和闭窗式两种，均可以用于单颗后牙种植修复。两种印模的制取难度都不大，最需要关注的是转移杆就位情况。只有完全就位的转移杆，才能制取准确的种植印模。

一般情况下，愈合基台、转移杆、修复基台穿龈部分的直径是相同的，只要愈合基台能够完全就位，它所对应的转移杆和修复基台就能就位。但也需要注意，同一个种植修复平台，可能会有不同直径的愈合基台、转移杆和修复基台，应使用同一直径的工具。如果使用了大直径的愈合基台，小直径的转移杆和修复基台可以就位；但如果使用小直径的愈合基

Physical impression

An implant level is commonly required to transfer the accurate position of the intraoral implant to the extraoral model. A transfer coping is connected to the implant and fixed inside the impression. After removing it from the mouth, the implant abutment is connected to an analogue of the implant, and then a gypsum model is poured.

1. Single posterior implant

Transfer copings are divided into open-tray and closed-tray types, both of which can be used for single posterior tooth implant restorations. The difficulty of making both types of impressions is not great, and the most important thing to pay attention to is the placement of the transfer coping. An accurate implant impression can only be taken with the transfer coping fully in place.

In general, the diameters of the healing abutments, transfer copings, and restorative abutments at the gingival level are the same. As long as the healing abutment can be fully seated, the corresponding transfer coping and restorative abutment can also be seated. However, it is important to note that for the same implant restoration platform, there may be healing abutments, transfer copings, and restorative abutments of different diameters, and tools of the same diameter should be used. If a larger diameter healing abutment is used, a smaller diameter transfer coping and restorative abutment can be seated; but if a smaller diameter healing abutment is used, there may be difficulty seating a larger

台，大直径的转移杆和修复基台可能会有就位困难。如果对于转移杆就位有疑虑，可以拍摄X线片进行确认。

制取开窗式印模的核心步骤是：试托盘大小合适→取下愈合基台并冲洗软组织袖口→连接开窗式转移杆并旋紧→托盘开窗→注入印模材料（一般是硅橡胶或者聚醚）→材料固化后旋松转移杆中央螺丝，取出印模→再次冲洗软组织袖口并安装愈合基台→开窗式转移杆连接种植体替代体。

制取闭窗式印模的核心步骤是：试托盘大小合适→取下愈合基台并冲洗软组织袖口→连接闭窗式转移杆并旋紧→注入印模材料（一般是硅橡胶或者聚醚）→材料固化后取出印模→取出闭窗式转移杆→再次冲洗软组织袖口并安装愈合基台→闭窗式转移杆连接种植体替代体→依靠闭窗式转移杆的特殊结构将其安插回印模上。

开窗式印模准确性相对较高，完全可以用于单颗后牙种植修复，但对开口度要求较高。闭窗式印模操作简便，其准确性也完全能满足单颗后牙种植修复的需求，在开口度不足的情况下，不失为一种实用的印模方式。

2. 单颗前牙

前牙种植修复除了要转移种植体位置信息以外，还需要复制过渡修复体的穿龈轮廓。前牙转移种植体位置的方式与后牙相同，但更推荐使用开窗式转移杆获得更准确的印模。前牙与后牙不同之处在于需要制作个性化转移杆，复制过渡修复体的穿龈轮廓。

diameter transfer coping and restorative abutment. If there is doubt about the proper seating of the transfer coping, X-rays is suggested to be taken for confirmation.

The core steps of making an open-tray impression include tray selection → removal of healing abutment and rinsing of soft tissue cuff → attachment and tightening of the open-tray transfer coping → windowing the tray → injecting impression material (usually silicone rubber or polyether) → releasing the central screw of the transfer coping after material curing, removing the impression → rinsing the soft tissue cuff again and installing the healing abutment → connecting the open-tray transfer coping to the implant analogue.

The core steps for making a closed-tray impression include the following: tray sizing → removal of the healing abutment and rinsing the soft tissue cuff → connecting the closed-tray transfer coping and tightening it → injecting the impression material (usually silicone rubber or polyether) → removing the impression after the material has set → removing the closed-tray transfer coping → rinsing the soft tissue cuff again and installing the healing abutment → connecting the implant analog with the closed-tray transfer coping → inserting it back in the impression using the special structure of the closed-tray transfer coping.

Open tray impression has relatively high accuracy and can be used for single posterior tooth implant restoration, but it requires higher opening width. Closed tray impression is easy to operate, and its accuracy can fully meet the needs of single posterior tooth implant restoration. In cases of narrow opening width, it is also a practical impression method.

2. Single anterior implant

Front tooth implant restoration not only requires transfer of implant position information, but also replication of the emergence profile of the interim restoration. The method of transferring implant position for front teeth is the same as for posterior teeth, but it is recommended to use an open-tray transfer coping to obtain a more accurate impression. The difference between anterior and posterior teeth lies in the necessity of fabricating a personalized transfer coping to replicate the emergence profile of the interim restoration.

取下过渡修复体后，种植体周围软组织袖口会逐渐收缩、塌陷，制取印模时即使在转移杆与软组织袖口之间注入印模材料也无法获取佩戴过渡修复体时软组织袖口的准确形态。按照过渡修复体穿龈轮廓制作个性化转移杆穿龈部分的形态，在灌制人工牙龈后可以得到软组织袖口的准确形态，为永久修复体复制过渡修复体穿龈轮廓提供准确的形态参考。

个性化转移杆制作方法如下：将过渡修复体连接到种植体替代体上→周围包裹一圈硅橡胶，覆盖全部穿龈轮廓但不超过外形高点→硅橡胶上标记唇侧面→取下过渡修复体→连接成品开窗转移杆→硅橡胶与转移杆的间隙中滴入收缩率低的化学固化材料，如成型树脂→材料固化后标记唇侧并取下转移杆→修整多余材料和锐利的边缘，完成个性化转移杆的制作。

3. 连续多颗种植体

连续多颗种植修复，无论是制作多个单冠，还是联冠或者固定桥，均建议采用开窗夹板式印模，最大限度提高各个种植体之间的位置关系准确性，保证修复体的被动就位。

牙线和流动树脂是临床常用的材料，但流动树脂的收缩比较大，在牙线上固化一段细长的流动树脂得到的强度较低，并不是特别理想的夹板方式。成型树脂的收缩比较小，也是修复常用材料，用它将金属杆连接到两个转移杆之间，可以获得较为坚固的夹板，是更推荐的夹板方式。金属杆可以专门制作，成本较低，也可以使用废旧车针代替。

After removing the interim restoration, the soft tissue cuff around the implant gradually shrinks and collapses. Even with impression material injected in the soft tissue cuff, it is difficult to obtain the accurate morphology of the soft tissue cuff when wearing the interim restoration. By creating a personalized transfer coping structure based on the emergence profile of the interim restoration, we can obtain the accurate morphology of the soft tissue cuff after casting the artificial gingiva. This process provides an accurate morphological reference for replicating the emergence profile of the interim restoration when fabricating the final prosthesis.

The method of personalized transfer coping production is as follows: connect the interim restoration to the implant abutment → wrap a ring of silicone rubber around it, covering the entire emergence profile but not exceeding the highest point of the outside shape → mark the buccal side on the silicone rubber → remove the interim restoration → connect the finished open-tray transfer coping → drop a low shrinkage chemical curing material, such as pattern resin, into the gap between the silicone rubber and the transfer coping → mark the labial side after the material is cured and remove the transfer coping → trim excess material and sharp edges to complete the production of a personalized transfer coping.

3. Continuous multiple implants

For continuous multiple restoration, whether making multiple single crowns, connecting crowns, or fixed bridges, it's recommended to use the open-tray impression technique to maximize the accuracy of the positional relationship between each implant and ensure the passive fit of the restoration.

Dental floss and flowable resin are commonly used materials in clinical practice. However, the shrinkage of flowable resin is relatively large. A long and thin section of flowable resin on dental floss results in lower strength is not an ideal splinting method. Pattern resin has smaller shrinkage and are also commonly used materials fin lab. By connecting a metal rod between two transfer copings using pattern resin, a stronger splint can be created, making it a more recommended method for splinting. The metal rod can be custom-made at a low cost or substituted with worn dental burs.

口内数字印模

种植修复的口内数字印模是通过扫描在种植体上连接的扫描杆，软件推算种植体位置。有些系统要求完整的扫描杆信息，有些系统原理上只需要扫描杆顶端的特殊结构信息就能计算出种植体位置。为了数据计算准确，建议数字印模中的扫描杆与牙槽嵴形成连续的三维图像，否则有些扫描软件可能会将游离的扫描杆顶部当作噪点自动删除，无法获得准确的扫描杆形态；穿出牙龈部分尽可能360°连续完整，不完整位置虽然会被软件自动补洞，但补洞未必是准确的，可能影响种植体位置的推算。

与物理印模中的转移杆一样，扫描杆也是需要完全就位，才能保证口内数字印模的准确性。常见的扫描杆材料有钛、聚醚醚酮（PEEK）、钛+PEEK。扫描杆的反复使用，可能会引起变形，影响就位，尤其是全PEEK扫描杆被施加扭力后，它与种植的接口容易发生变形。钛或者钛+PEEK扫描杆的基底部分是金属材质，相对不容易变形，但也应该在出厂说明所允许的使用次数内，且不宜施加过大扭力。

1. 单颗后牙

单颗后牙种植修复需要制取的数字印模十分简便，通常仅需要4个扫描文件：工作颌牙列（包含种植体周围牙龈袖口、近远中至少一颗邻牙）、扫描杆、对颌牙列、咬合信息（图22~图25）。一般情况下，扫描杆信息是在工作颌牙列数据中补扫而得，无需重新扫描牙列，也不要求扫描杆数字印模中的邻牙形态完整。

Intraoral digital impression

Intraoral digital impressions of the implants are calculated by scanning the scan post connected to the implant and inferring the position of the implant. Most systems require complete information of the scan post, while other a few theoretically only need the special structural information at the top of the scan post to calculate the position of the implant. For accurate data calculation, it is recommended that the scan post in the digital impression forms a continuous three-dimensional image with the alveolar ridge. Otherwise, some scanning software may automatically delete the free scan post tops as noise, resulting in inaccurate scan post morphology. The gingival portion should be as complete as possible to have a continuous, 360° image. Although incomplete areas will be automatically filled by the software, the filled areas may not be accurate and may affect the calculation of the implant position.

Just as in physical transfer copings, scan posts need to be fully seated to ensure the accuracy of intraoral digital impressions. Common materials for scan posts include titanium, PEEK, and titanium + PEEK. Repeated use of scan posts may cause deformation, affecting seating. This is especially true when full PEEK scan posts are subjected to torque, as they are prone to deformation at the implant interface. The base portion of titanium or titanium + PEEK scan posts is made of metal and is relatively less prone to deformation. However, it should still be used within the allowed number of uses stated in the manufacturer's instructions, and excessive torque should be avoided.

1. Single posterior implant

The digital impression for single posterior implant restoration is very simple to create, typically requiring only four scans: working dentition (including the emergence profile around the implant, adjacent teeth in the mesial and distal), scan posts, opposing dentition, and bite information (Figs. 22 to 25). Generally, the scan post information is obtained by rescanning the working dentition, without the need to rescan the entire dentition, and without the requirement for complete morphology of adjacent teeth in the scan post digital impression.

蜕变——数字化种植导板与全瓷修复中的医技实践
Metamorphosis: Clinical and Technological Practices in Digital Surgical Templates and Ceramic Restorations for Implants

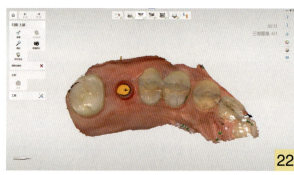

22 工作颌牙列数字印模
Working dentition

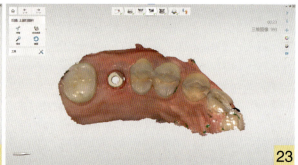

23 扫描杆数字印模
Scan post

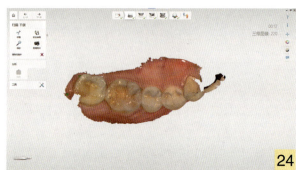

24 对颌牙列数字印模
Opposing dentition

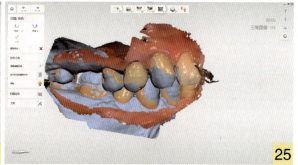

25 颊侧数字印模
Buccal side scanning for occlusion

2. 单颗前牙

前牙种植修复的口内数字印模也需要复制过渡修复体穿龈轮廓，有直接扫描软组织袖口和口外扫描过渡修复体两种方式可供参考。

（1）直接扫描软组织袖口。虽然取下过渡修复体后，软组织袖口会发生收缩、塌陷，但在刚取下修复体的时候，其变化较小，对美学效果影响较小。如果可以在取下修复体短时间内（一般不超过10秒）记录软组织袖口形态，则可以简便地复制过渡修复体穿龈轮廓。

2. Single anterior implant

The intraoral digital impression of anterior teeth implant restoration also needs to replicate the emergence profile of the interim restoration, with two reference options available: direct scanning of soft tissue cuff in the mouth and scanning of the interim restoration outside the mouth.

(1) Direct scanning of soft tissue cuff in the mouth. Although the soft tissue cuff will shrink and collapse after removing the interim restoration, the changes are minimal in a very short time, resulting in minimal impact on the aesthetic effect. If the soft tissue cuff morphology can be recorded shortly after removing the restoration (generally within 10 seconds), the interim

口内数字印模的补扫功能，可以实现数秒内完成单颗种植体软组织袖口形态采集（图26~图29）。

（2）口外扫描过渡修复体（图30~图35）。此方法需要6个印模数据：①制取戴过渡修复体的牙列数字印模；②取下过渡修复体，补扫邻牙邻面；③扫描杆；④对颌牙列；⑤咬合扫描；⑥将过渡修复体在口外单独进行扫描，获得完整清楚的牙冠及穿龈轮廓。

restoration emergence profile can be easily replicated. The supplemental scanning function of intraoral digital impressions can quickly collect the morphology of the soft tissue cuff around a single implant in a matter of seconds (Figs. 26 to 29).

(2) Scanning of the interim restoration outside the mouth (Figs. 30 to 35). This method requires 6 template data: ①Dentition wearing the interim restoration; ②Remove the interim restoration and scan the adjacent tooth surfaces; ③Scan post; ④The opposing dentition; ⑤Occlusal relation; ⑥Scan the transition repair group outside the mouth separately to obtain a complete and clear contour including the emergence profile.

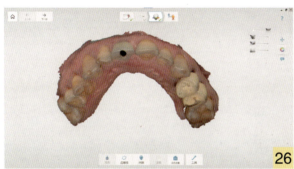

26　戴过渡修复体的牙列
Dentition with interim restorations

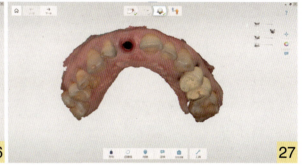

27　补扫穿龈轮廓
Soft tissue cuff refinement

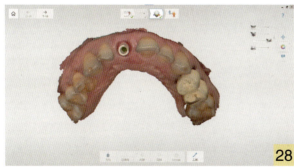

28　扫描杆数字印模
Scan post

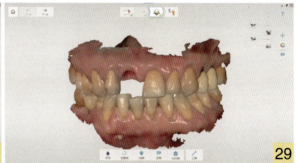

29　对颌及咬合
Opposing dentition and occlusal relationship

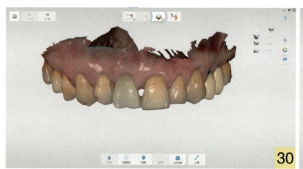

30 戴过渡修复体的牙列
Dentition with interim restoration

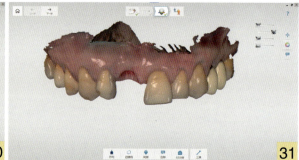

31 补扫邻牙邻面
Adjacent teeth

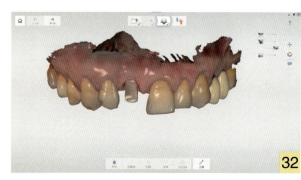

32 补扫扫描杆
Scan post

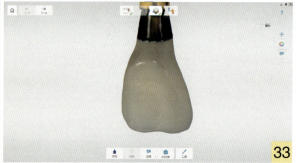

33 过渡修复体数字印模
The interim restoration

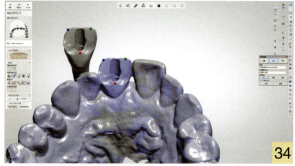

34 对齐修复体与牙列数字印模
Alignment of the restoration with dentition

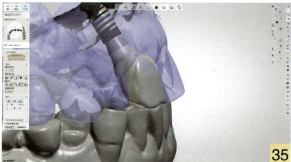

35 完成修复体设计
Completion of restoration design

永久修复体设计时可以将数据⑥与数据①配准，这样在设计穿龈轮廓时可以直接复制过渡修复体的穿龈轮廓，并不直接参考牙龈袖口形态。因此，采用这种方式时即使牙龈袖口形态变化了，也不影响修复体制作。

3. 连续多颗种植体

口内数字印模并不需要用夹板固定扫描杆，确保每个扫描杆都被准确、清晰地扫描即可（图36和图37）。然而，由于口内数字印模系统扫描黏膜的能力相对较弱，因此当跨越较大范围黏膜时，印模的准确性会下降。通常，3个以上种植体或者超过5单位的联冠或者固定桥，使用口内数字印模制作修复体获得良好被动就位的难度较大。

During the design of a definitive restoration, data ⑥ can be registered with data ①, allowing the contour of the interim restoration to be directly copied during the design of the emergence profile, instead of referencing the soft tissue morphology. Therefore, using this method, changes in the soft tissue cuff do not affect the fabrication of the restoration.

3. Continuous multiple implants

Intraoral digital impressions do not require the splinting the scan posts, but ensuring that each post is scanned accurately and clearly (Figs. 36 and 37). However, due to the relatively weak ability of intraoral digital impression systems to scan mucosa, the accuracy of the impression will decrease when scanning a large area of mucosa. Typically, difficulties in obtaining a well-fitting prosthesis with good passive fit arise when making restorations using intraoral digital impressions with 3 or more implants, or more than 5 units of implant-supported fixed bridge.

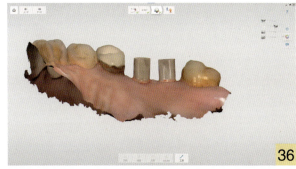

36 种植联冠修复体数字印模
Digital impression of multiple united crowns

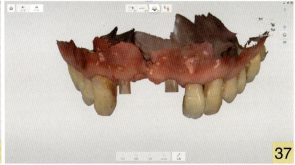

37 种植固定桥数字印模
Impression of fixed bridge

牙列缺损种植修复体的设计

当技师拿到带有种植体位置信息和轮廓信息的印模时，就可以开始修复体设计，需确定修复体的固位形式、结构类型、材料选择等，虽然在本节才讨论这些内容，但实际上理应在治疗前就有明确的计划。

1. 固位形式

修复体的主要固位形式有螺丝固位和粘接固位两类，两类修复体各有优缺点，临床工作中两种固位形式的修复体都可能会用到。

螺丝固位临床操作简单，对于轴向较好的单冠、种植体之间夹角较小的联冠或固定桥，都建议采取螺丝固位。螺丝固位修复体就位时基台与种植体、基台与软组织袖口、牙冠与邻牙等多处都发生接触，需要这些接触位置都同时、刚好发生合适力度的接触，对加工的准确性要求较高。螺丝固位修复体在戴牙时，对开口度要求较高，但对咬合间隙的需求相对较小。

粘接固位最大的缺点是多余粘接剂的残留可能会增加种植体周围炎的风险，为了便于粘接剂的清除，修复体边缘位置最好不深于龈下0.5mm。其次是临床粘接可能会有唾液污染粘接界面，降低粘接力。但粘接固位对种植体轴向的宽容度较大。如果前牙区螺丝孔穿出点位于唇侧或者切缘，螺丝固位会影响美观效果，则建议采用粘接固位。如果多个种植体之间的夹角较大，制作螺丝固位的联冠或者固定桥，被动就位的难度较大，可以考虑使用个性化或

Section three design of implant restorations for defected dentition

When the technician receives the impression containing the position information and contour information of the implant, they can start designing the prosthesis, determining the form of prosthesis fixation, structural type, material selection, etc. Although these topics are discussed in this section after surgery, there should be a clear plan before the treatment.

1. Fixed form

The main fixed forms of dental restorations are screw fixation and adhesive fixation, each of which has its own advantages and disadvantages. Both types of fixed restorations may be used in clinical practice.

Screw retention is simple in clinical operation, and screw retention is recommended for single crowns with good axial alignment, interproximal angles between implants, or fixed bridges with small angles. When the screw-retained restoration is in place, there are multiple points of contact, such as the abutment - the implant, the abutment - the soft tissue cuff, and the crown - the adjacent teeth, all of which require appropriate and simultaneous contact. This requires a high level of accuracy in fabrication. When wearing a screw-retained restoration, a high degree of mouth opening is required, but the demand for occlusal clearance is relatively small.

The main disadvantage of adhesive fixation is that the residue of excess adhesive may increase the risk of inflammation around the implant. In order to facilitate the removal of the adhesive, it is better for the margin of the restoration not to be deeper than 0.5mm below the gingival margin. Secondly, clinical bonding may have saliva contamination at the bonding interface, reducing the bonding strength. However, the tolerance of adhesive fixation to the axial direction of the implant is larger. If the screw hole in the anterior area exits on the labial side or the incisal edge and screw fixation affects the aesthetic outcome, it is recommended to use adhesive fixation. If the angle between multiple implants is large, making a screw fixation bridge between them is challenging in passive fit. In this case, consider using customized or prefabricated angled abutments to provide a common

者成品的角度基台提供共同就位道，采用粘接固位形式固定联冠或者固定桥。粘接固位修复体的基台与冠部结构是分开就位的，加工的宽容度相对较大。粘接固位修复体可以用于开口度更小的情况，但需要更大的咬合间隙。

2. 结构类型

传统的种植修复体由基台和冠两部分组成。如果是不需要制作个性化的穿龈轮廓的情况，无论螺丝固位还是粘接固位，成品基台＋冠这种结构在临床的应用都十分常见。如果需要制作个性化穿龈轮廓，且固位形式是粘接固位，则建议使用单层材料（一般是金属钛）的个性化基台，再粘接冠修复体，可用于后牙或者黏膜较厚不会透出基台颜色的前牙。

随着粘接技术的提高，修复材料性能的改善，钛基底（Ti-Base）的应用逐渐成熟。Ti-Base+瓷材料制作修复体，可以很好地满足个性化的穿龈轮廓、避免牙龈颜色变深两个要求。如果是粘接固位，可以采用Ti-Base制作个性化瓷基台，再粘接冠修复体，但需要保证每层材料都有足够厚度（图38）；如果是螺丝固位，可以在Ti-Base上制作个性化基台一体冠，修复体的设计与制作更加简便（图39）。

单层材料的个性化基台一体冠也有一定的临床意义。当遇到咬合间隙特别小的情况，可以采用单层材料的个性化基台一体冠，理论上只要能容纳修复螺丝的空间，就能容纳此类修复体。然而，在设计修复体时才发现咬合间隙不足，是一种不正确的临床行为，理应在种植治疗开始之前就评估咬合间隙，如果间隙不够

path for positioning, and cement the bridge. The abutment and crown structure of the adhesive fixation restoration are positioned separately, with relatively large tolerance in fabrication. Adhesive fixation restoration can be used in cases with a smaller opening, but a larger occlusal gap is required.

2. Structural type

The traditional implant restoration consists of the abutment and crown. In cases where personalized emergence profiles are not required, whether screw-retained or cement-retained, the combination of prefabricated abutment and crown is commonly used in clinical practice. For cases requiring personalized emergence profiles and cement-retained restorations, it is recommended to use a personalized abutment made from a single layer material (usually titanium alloy), followed by the cementation of the crown. This type of restoration can be used on posterior teeth or anterior teeth with thick mucosa that does not allow the abutment color to show through.

With the improvement of adhesive technology and the enhancement of repair material performance, the application of titanium base (Ti-Base) is gradually maturing. Ti-Base combined with ceramic material can meet the requirements of personalized emergence profile and prevent gingival color darkening. When using adhesive fixation, personalized ceramic abutments can be made with Ti-Base, followed by adhesive crown restorations. It is necessary to ensure that each layer of material has sufficient thickness (Fig. 38). For screw fixation, a personalized abutment-crown can be made in one piece on the Ti-Base, making the design and fabrication of the restoration more convenient (Fig. 39).

The individualized abutment-crown monoblock of single-layer material also has certain clinical significance. When facing situations with very small occlusal gaps, the individualized abutment-crown monoblock of single-layer material can be used. In theory, as long as there is enough space to accommodate the repair screw, this type of repair can be accommodated. However, it is an incorrect clinical behavior to discover insufficient occlusal clearance only when designing the restoration. Occlusal clearance should be evaluated before implant

应该考虑通过正畸压低对颌牙、调磨对颌牙、抬高咬合等方法创造足够的咬合间隙，而不是到设计修复体时进行弥补。

3. 材料选择

基台材料最常见的是金属钛，用于薄龈型前牙可能会透出金属颜色，使牙龈颜色发灰发暗，影响美学效果。单纯氧化锆基台现在应用较少，种植体接口部位的基台较薄，氧化锆用在该处发生折断的风险较高。但可以使用Ti-Base和氧化锆两种材料共同组成基台，既能保证强度，也不会导致牙龈颜色变灰变暗。Ti-Base和聚醚醚酮（polyether-ether-ketone，PEEK）也可以制作修复基台，同时具备良好的机械性能和美学效果（图40）。

treatment begins. If the clearance is insufficient, methods such as orthodontic leveling of opposing teeth, grinding of opposing teeth, and increasing vertical dimension should be considered to create enough occlusal clearance, rather than trying to compensate at the time of designing the restoration.

3. Material selection

The most common material for abutments is titanium. This material may cause the metal color to show through in thin gingival-type anterior teeth, resulting in the gingival color turning gray and dark, which can affect the aesthetic effect. Pure zirconia abutments are currently less used because the abutment at the implant interface is thin, leading to a higher risk of zirconia fracture in that area. However, a combination of Ti-Base and zirconia can be used for the abutment, which can ensure strength and avoid the gingival color turning gray or dark. Ti-Base with pressed polyether-ether-ketone (PEEK) can also be used to fabricate restorative abutments, providing good mechanical properties and aesthetic effects simultaneously (Fig. 40).

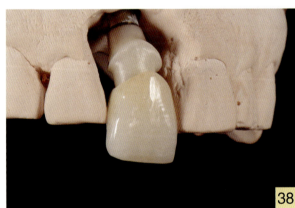

38 Ti-Base个性化氧化锆基台粘接固位冠
Ti-Base customized zirconia abutment with bonded crown

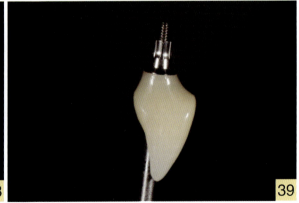

39 Ti-Base个性化氧化锆基台一体冠
Ti-Base customized zirconia abutment-crown

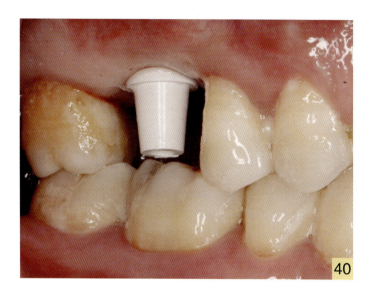

40　PEEK基台
　　PEEK abutment

冠修复体材料从铸造金属、金属烤瓷，发展至今越来越常见的是全瓷材料。单层高透渐变色氧化锆可以满足多数情况的美学需求和强度要求，是非常好的冠修复体材料。对于美学要求特别高的情况，氧化锆基底外部烤瓷可以呈现极好的美学效果。二硅酸锂增强型玻璃陶瓷在种植修复中也有应用，它的强度和美学效果介于氧化锆和烤瓷之间。

本书第4章将详细介绍各种常见的种植修复全瓷材料，医生、技师需要熟悉材料性能，根据临床具体条件选择合适的材料。

牙列缺损种植修复体的试戴与随访

如果前面的种植外科治疗完善，印模精准，修复体设计合理、加工准确，修复体戴牙会非常顺利，并不会有太高难度。

The materials for crown restorations have evolved from casting metals, metal-ceramics, to the increasingly common all-ceramic materials. A single layer of high translucent gradient color zirconia can meet most aesthetic and strength requirements, making it a very good crown restoration material. For cases with particularly high aesthetic requirements, external porcelain baking on a zirconia base can achieve excellent aesthetic effects. Lithium disilicate reinforced glass ceramic is also used in implant restorations, with its strength and aesthetic effects falling between zirconia and porcelain.

Chapter 4 of this book details various common planting repairs for all-ceramic materials. Doctors and technicians need to be familiar with the material properties and select suitable materials based on specific clinical conditions.

Section four delivery and follow-up

If the previous planting surgery is well done, the impression is accurate, the prosthesis design is reasonable, and the processing is accurate, the delivery of the restoration will be very smooth without too much difficulty.

修复体的被动就位是首先需要关注的。螺丝固位修复体是整体同时就位的，根据修复体形态和螺丝方向，可以引导修复体就位；粘接固位修复体基台与冠分开就位，一般会使用成型树脂制作或者树脂3D打印一个小工具，通过邻牙引导修复基台正确就位。修复体就位后非常有必要拍摄X线片，确定就位完全。

种植体与天然牙对咬合力量的反应并不相同。天然牙受到垂直向咬合力量时，在垂直向运动幅度可达25～100μm，种植体只有3～5μm；受侧向力时，二者在水平向的运动幅度差异更大。有一种观点是种植修复体"轻咬不接触，重咬轻接触"，然而这个"轻"与"重"并没有明确指标，种植体与天然牙生理动度的差异并非固定不变。临床上很难精确做到理论上最理想的状态，但适当降低种植体的秴力负担是值得考虑的。同时也警惕过于奔放的调秴方式，使得种植修复体的咬合完全被调空，无法提供有效的咬合作用。

戴牙并不是种植修复的终点，定期随访有助于及时发现并解决问题，提高种植治疗的长期成功率。戴牙1～2周后复查口腔卫生维护情况；1个月后检查咬合状态；之后每6～12个月检查软硬组织稳定性。由于修复体磨耗速度低于天然牙，随访过程中应注意修复体的咬合负担是否变重。大量临床研究都发现了种植修复体的邻接触丧失，因此每次随访还应注意邻接触是否有变松，尤其是近中邻面，必要时需要对修复体进行加瓷处理。

The passive placement of the restoration is the first thing to focus on. Screw-retained restorations are seated as a whole, guiding the restoration into place based on the morphology of the restoration and the screw direction. Adhesive-retained restorations have the abutment and crown seated separately. Generally, a small tool made of pattern resin or 3D printed resin will be used to guide the abutment into the correct position through the adjacent teeth. It is very necessary to take X-rays after the restoration is seated to confirm complete placement.

The response of implants to occlusal forces is different from natural teeth. When subjected to vertical occlusal forces, natural teeth can move vertically up to 25-100μm, while implants only move 3-5μm. The difference in horizontal movement under lateral forces is even greater between the two. There is a view that implants should have "no contact on light bites, and light contact on heavy bites", but the terms "light" and "heavy" lack clear criteria, and the difference in physiological mobility between implants and natural teeth is not always the same. In clinical practice, achieving the theoretically ideal state is difficult, but it is worth considering properly reducing the load on implants. At the same time, caution should be exercised against overly aggressive occlusal adjustments, which may result in the occlusion of implant restorations being completely disregarded, leading to ineffective occlusal function.

Delivery is not the end of implant treatment. Regular follow-up visits help to timely detect and solve problems, improving the long-term success rate of implant treatment. Recheck oral hygiene maintenance 1-2 weeks after wearing dentures; check occlusal status after 1 month, and then check the stability of soft and hard tissues every 6-12 months. Due to the low wear rate of the restoration compared to natural teeth, during follow-up, attention should be paid to whether the bite burden of the restoration has increased. Many clinical studies have found that loss of adjacent contact of implant restorations is a common issue. Therefore, it is necessary to pay attention to whether adjacent contact has become loose during each follow-up, especially focusing on the mesial contact. Ceramic addition to the restoration may be necessary in case of the loss of proximal contact.

全牙列种植固定修复的基本流程与技术要点

PROCEDURAL AND TECHNICAL ESSENTIALS OF FULL ARCH IMPLANT-SUPPORTED FIXED PROSTHESES

全牙列种植治疗与牙列缺损种植冠桥修复有不同的即刻负重需求和修复理念。虽然分段式固定桥也是全牙列固定修复的一种方式，但二级螺丝固定的一体式桥架更容易实现被动就位，有广泛的临床应用，本章将对后者展开详细讨论。

The immediate loading requirements and restorative concepts for full-arch implant treatment differ from those for fixed bridge restorations of missing dental arches. While segmented fixed bridges are an option for full-arch fixed restorations, frameworks secured with secondary screws are more commonly used in clinical practice due to their easier achievement of passive fit. This chapter will provide an in-depth discussion on the latter approach.

第1节　全牙列种植即刻过渡修复

Section 1 Immediate Interim Restorations for Full Arch Implants

印模制取与颌位关系记录

Impression and maxillo-mandibular relationship recording

全牙列种植的患者在术后往往没有余留牙提供咀嚼功能，对即刻负重的需求较大，种植体需要有良好的初期稳定性，即刻过渡修复体应满足即刻负重的要求。种植术中根据种植体角度选择合适的复合基台，尽量使各个复合基台二级螺丝方向平行，但并不要求完全平行，再安装牙龈保护帽，关闭伤口（图1），拍片确认种植体位置良好、复合基台完全就位后则开始即刻修复。

Patients undergoing full arch implantation often have no remaining teeth to provide masticatory function post-surgery, thus necessitating immediate loading. The implants must be in good initial stability, and the immediate transitional prosthesis should accommodate the requirements for immediate loading. During surgery, appropriate multi-unit abutments are selected based on the implant angle, aiming to align the directions of the secondary screws of each multi-unit abutment as parallel as possible, though complete parallelism was not required. Subsequently, the gingival protective caps are screwed, and the wound is sutured (Fig. 1). After radiographic confirmation that the implants are correctly positioned and the multi-unit abutments are fully seated, immediate loading commences.

印模水平为基台水平印模。关键操作步骤如下：在复合基台上连接转移杆并拧紧（图2），拍摄曲面体层片或根尖片确定转移杆完全就位（图3）→再使用成型树脂和金属杆连接各个转移杆（图4），保证转移杆之间的相互位置准确→试戴并选择大小合适的成品托盘，在各转移杆对应的托盘位置开孔→使用硅橡胶制取印模→硅橡胶固化后拧松转移杆，取出印模（图5）→转移杆上连接复合基台替代体。

Typically, abutment-level impressions are utilized. The key procedural steps are as follows: First, connect the transfer copings to the multi-unit abutments tightly (Fig. 2) and X-ray examination is required to ensure the copings are in right positions (Fig. 3). Next, use pattern resin and metal copings to connect each transfer coping (Fig. 4), ensuring precise alignment of the transfer copings. Select and try the appropriate size of the impression tray and create openings at the positions corresponding to each transfer coping. Use silicone rubber to create the impression. Once the silicone rubber has set, loosen the transfer copings, and remove the impression (Fig. 5). Finally, reconnect the analogues in place of the transfer copings.

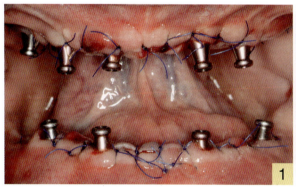

1　安装牙龈保护帽缝合完成后
Sutures following gingival protective caps screwed

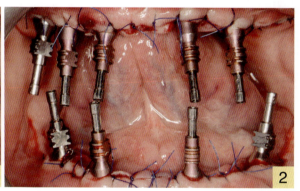

2　安装复合基台转移杆
Installation of multi-unit abutment transfer copings

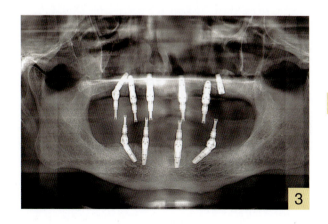

3　安装复合基台转移杆拍摄曲面体层片
Panoramic photography after installation of transfer copings

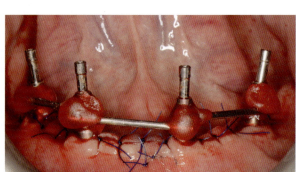 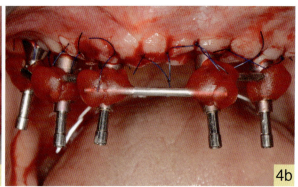

4 口内连接转移杆
Intraoral connection transfer copings

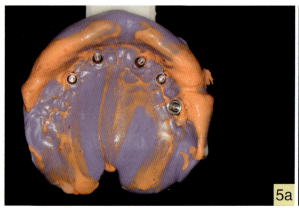 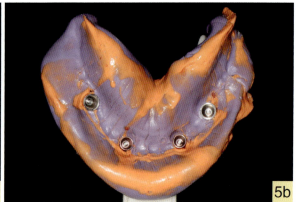

5 全口种植修复印模
Silicone impressions

复合基台位于龈下过深的位置，会增加转移杆就位的难度。全口种植修复的转移杆不推荐使用牙线+流动树脂制作夹板固定，该夹板稳定性不足，转移杆之间仍然容易发生移位或倾斜。

颌位关系记录包括正中关系和垂直距离两部分；如果有上颌修复，还应标记牙中线和𬌗平面。灌制模型后制作暂基托和蜡堤，再进行颌位关系记录，是最稳妥的方式。但有时候为了提高临床效率，有经验的医生也可以使用固

The multi-unit abutment should not be positioned too deeply, which complicates the placement of the transfer coping. For full-arch implant restorations, it's not recommended to use dental floss combined with flowable resin to create a splint for securing the transfer coping due to insufficient stability, leading to potential displacement or tilting of the transfer copings.

Recording occlusal relationships involves capturing centric relation and vertical dimension; for maxillary rehabilitation, the tooth midline and incisal plane should also be marked. The most reliable method is to create a temporary base and wax rims after model pouring, followed by recording the occlusal relationships. However, experienced clinicians may opt to use fast-

化速度较快的硅橡胶直接在患者口内确定颌位关系。

通过立体摄影测量技术获取种植体位置信息，与口内数字印模配准，可以制取全口种植的数字印模，但颌位记录还需要制作暂基托和蜡堤，或者通过CT配准术前的咬合关系。全程种植导板引导下不翻瓣手术，可以术前制作过渡修复体，术后连接临时钛基底后重衬过渡修复体。在合适的条件下，这两种数字化方式也是良好的临床选择，但本章内容主要还是着重于物理印模，这是目前较容易开展的方式。

技工室制作

技师拿到印模之后，先对印模进行清洁消毒，一般采用浸泡消毒方式。再确定转移杆位置稳定，不易移动，复合基台替代体完全就位于转移杆上，并且转移杆螺丝已旋紧。接着在转移杆和替代体颈部注射人工牙龈，灌制石膏模型，上𬭚架。

然后将临时钛基底安装在替代体上（图6），根据咬合间隙调整临时钛基底的长度。再把厚度和宽度都足够的金属条弯制成合适形态，与所有临时钛基底连接在一起，形成修复体的支架，以保证戴牙后种植体之间都是刚性连接，并增强过渡义齿的强度（图7）。在支架上排牙，制作蜡型，注塑，打磨抛光（图8～图10）。将完成的过渡修复体消毒后再转回临床（图11）。随着材料性能的提升，熟练的技师接到印模和颌位记录后只需2小时左右就能完成全牙列即刻过渡修复体的制作。

curing silicone rubber to directly determine occlusal relationships in the patient's mouth, thereby enhancing clinical efficiency.

Using stereophotogrammetry technology, the positional information of implants can be obtained and registered with intraoral digital impressions to produce a comprehensive digital impression of full-mouth implants. Nevertheless, the jaw relationship record must still be captured using either a temporary base and wax dam or through CT registration of the preoperative jaw relationship. Flapless surgery fully guided by a template enables to use the preoperative fabrication of transitional restorations, which can then be connected to temporary titanium abutments and re-lined postoperatively. Under appropriate conditions, both digital approaches offer viable clinical options. However, this chapter primarily focuses on physical impressions, which remain an accessible and effective method.

Laboratory procedure

After the technician receives the impression, the first step is to clean and disinfect the impression, usually by soaking. Then, ensure that the transfer copings are stable and not easily moved, the analogues are in place on the transfer copings tightly. Next, inject artificial gingiva at the neck of the transfer copings and analogues, pour the gypsum model, and set it on the articulator.

Then install the temporary titanium base on the abutment (Fig. 6), adjust the length of the temporary titanium base according to the occlusal space. Then bend metal strips with sufficient thickness and width into the appropriate shape, connect it on to the temporary titanium bases to form the framework of the restoration, to ensure a rigid connection between the implants after wearing, and to enhance the strength of the restoration (Fig. 7). Arrange teeth on the framework, make a wax pattern, injection molding, and polish (Figs. 8 to 10). After disinfecting the completed interim restoration, return it to the clinic (Fig. 11). With the improvement of material performance, proficient technicians who receive the impression and jaw relation record only need about 2 hours to complete the fabrication of immediate interim restorations for full arch.

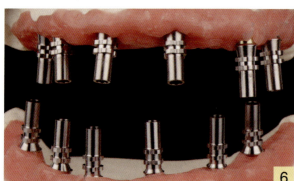

6 安装钛基底
Installation of titanium bases

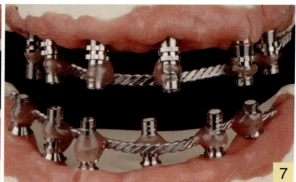

7 连接钛条
Connection of titanium bar

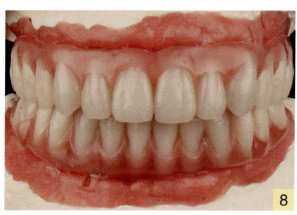

8 制作蜡型
Making the wax pattern

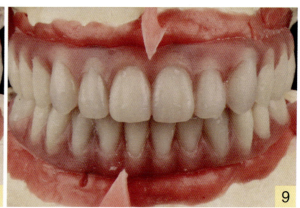

9 注塑完成
Injection molding completed

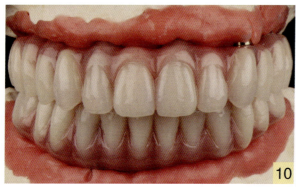

10 抛光后的修复体
Polished restoration

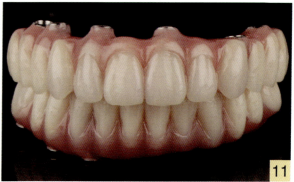

11 修复体完成
Restoration completed

戴牙与随访

最好能在手术当天或者24小时内完成戴牙，随着术后时间的增加，牙槽嵴肿胀增加，会妨碍过渡修复体就位。牙槽嵴消肿需要1~2周的时间，等待时间过长也有悖于即刻负重的初衷，长时间没有过渡修复体，患者可能会用某一两颗种植体上的牙龈保护帽进行咬合，对种植体是非常危险的受力方式。

戴牙时，必须确认过渡修复体的被动就位。戴入时的手感可以帮助医生判断就位情况；拍摄曲面体层片或根尖片，进一步明确修复体的就位情况（图12和图13）。

确认修复体就位后，需暂封螺丝孔，检查咬合状态，并调𬌗至正中𬌗均匀接触，非正中𬌗无干扰，螺丝孔附近修复体较薄的位置可以适当减轻咬合接触。

术后3天复查伤口初步愈合情况，有无出血，有无感染；2周复查软组织愈合情况，拆除缝线，检查口腔卫生，检查咬合并进行必要的调𬌗；之后1个月复查一次，检查并确保口腔卫生和咬合均处于良好的状态。

Delivery and follow-up

The restoration should ideally be inserted on the day of surgery or within 24 hours. Delaying the insertion leads to increased swelling of the alveolar ridge, which complicates the placement of the prosthetic device. Typically, it takes 1-2 weeks for the swelling of the alveolar ridge to subside. Prolonged waiting is counterproductive to the concept of immediate loading. If the interim restoration is not placed promptly, the patient might use the gingival protection cap on one or two dental implants to occlude, posing a significant risk to the implants.

While delivery, it is crucial to confirm the passive fit. The tactile feedback during insertion assists the dentist in assessing the fit; radiographs should be taken to further verify the positioning of the restoration (Figs. 12 and 13).

After confirming the restoration is in place, temporarily seal the screw holes, check the occlusion, adjust the contact to the even distribution in central occlusion, without interference in non-central occlusion, and appropriately reduce the occlusal contact at the thinner position near the screw hole.

A postoperative checkup should be conducted 3 days after surgery to assess the initial wound healing and to check for bleeding and infection. Two weeks later, a follow-up is required to review the healing of soft tissues, remove stitches, evaluate oral hygiene, and assess occlusion, making necessary adjustments. Subsequently, monthly follow-ups should be scheduled to ensure proper oral hygiene and occlusion.

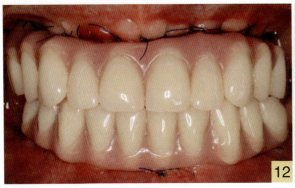

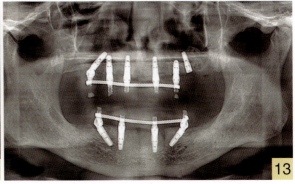

12 戴即刻过渡修复体
The insertion of immediate interim restorations

13 戴修复体拍摄曲面体层片
Panoramic radiograph after the insertion

第2节 全牙列种植永久固定修复

Section 2 Definitive Fixed Restorations for Full Arch Implants

印模制取与颌位记录

制取印模前，在制作过渡修复体的模型上安装转移杆，并使用成型树脂制作夹板连接所有的转移杆，并断开连接以释放应力。在安装转移杆的模型上制作个别托盘。

过渡义齿在过渡期使用良好，咬合稳定，颌位关系正确，则可以利用过渡义齿转移颌位记录，将模型上𬌗架（图14和图15）。如果需要重新确定颌位关系，则应制作暂基托、蜡堤，哥特式弓确定颌位关系（图16）。

使用面弓转移上颌位置。

制取印模时，先要给复合基台加力，确保一级螺丝的扭矩达到了35Ncm。然后按顺序在患者口内安装这些带着成型树脂夹板的转移杆（图17），拍摄X线片确认转移杆就位（图18），把夹板断开处使用成型树脂再次连接（图19）。这种方式可以最大限度降低夹板中的应力，提高种植体之间位置的准确度。使用个别托盘和流动性较好的硅橡胶或者聚醚制取印模，记录准确的种植体位置和牙槽嵴形态（图20）。

Impression and maxillo-mandibular relationship recording

Before taking impressions, attach the transfer posts to the model for creating the interim restoration, and use pattern resin to section all the transfer posts, then disconnect them to relieve stress. Fabricate individual trays on the model with the attached transfer posts.

During the transitional phase, if the interim restoration is functioning well, occlusion is stable, and the jaw relationship is correct, the interim restoration can be used to transfer the jaw relationship to articulate the models (Figs. 14 and 15). If it is necessary to re-establish the jaw relationship, utilize a temporary baseplate, wax rims, and a Gothic arch to determine the jaw relationship (Fig. 16).

Using a facebow to transfer the maxillary position.

When taking impressions, initially apply a force to the multi-unit abutments to ensure that the primary screws reach a torque of 35Ncm. Then sequentially install these transfer copings with pattern resin splints in the patient's mouth (Fig. 17), take X-rays to confirm the position of the transfer copings (Fig. 18), and reconnect the trays at the break points using pattern resin (Fig. 19). This method can minimize stress among the posts and improve accuracy in the positioning of the implants. Use individual trays and silicone or polyether to take impressions, recording the accurate positions of the implants and alveolar ridge morphology (Fig. 20).

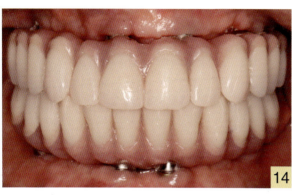

14 功能状态良好的过渡修复体
Interim restoration with good functional status

15 过渡修复体咬合记录
Occlusal records by interim restorations

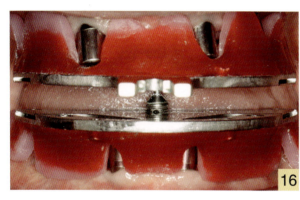

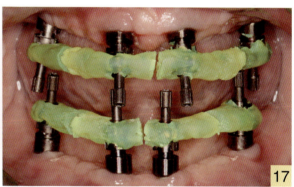

16 哥特式弓确定颌位关系
Jaw relation recording by a Gothic arch

17 安装转移杆
Installation of transfer copings

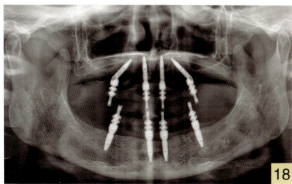

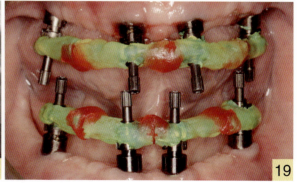

18 拍摄曲面体层片
Panoramic photography

19 转移杆夹板再连接
Reconnection of transfer copings

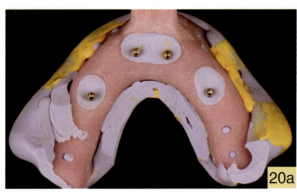
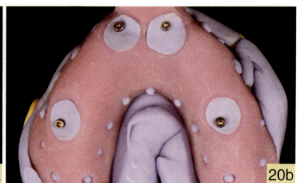

20 硅橡胶印模
Silicone impressions

技工室制作

技师拿到印模后灌制模型，将模型上𬌗架（图21和图22），参考过渡修复体形态为永久修复体排牙，制作的蜡型称为评估桥。在患者口内试戴评估桥，评估正中关系是否正确，垂直距离是否合适，𬌗平面是否正确，外观是否满足美学要求（图23和图24）。若完全不需修改，技师则按照评估桥形态制作永久修复体；若需要少量修改，技师可以立即修改后再给患者试戴；若需要大量修改，则可能带回技工室修改好后再次预约患者试戴更好。

钛桥架加全瓷外冠是目前最常用的修复体结构。确认评估桥形态无需再修改后，技师扫描评估桥，复制其外形，牙冠部分和唇颊侧牙龈形态作为永久修复体相应部位的形态，舌侧牙龈部分可以适当修薄，减少舌侧体积，减小

Laboratory procedure

After receiving the impression, the technician pours the model and places it on the articulator (Figs. 21 and 22). They refer to the transitional restoration form as the definitive restoration form and create a wax pattern known as an evaluation bridge. The patient then tries on the evaluation bridge to assess the centric relation, vertical dimension, occlusal plane, and aesthetic appearance (Figs. 23 and 24). If no modifications are required, the technician proceeds to fabricate the definitive restoration based on the evaluation bridge. If minor adjustments are needed, the technician can make them immediately and have the patient try it on again. For major modifications, the technician may need to return the bridge to the laboratory for adjustments before scheduling another appointment for the patient to try it on again.

The combination of a titanium framework and all-ceramic crowns is currently the most used restorative structure. Once the bridge form has been confirmed and evaluated without the need for further modifications, the technician scans and assesses the bridge, replicating its shape, the tooth crown portion, and the labial and buccal

患者的异物感。得到永久修复体外形后，回切全瓷牙冠和唇颊侧牙龈烤塑的空间，就得到了钛桥架的形态。

钛桥架加工之前，还可以用PMMA加工一个桥架（图25），验证设计数据是否合理，加工设备是否准确。一切验证妥当后，再切削钛桥架（图26）。在𬌗架上试戴桥架的就位情况和外冠的修复空间。然后钛桥架需要遮色（图27），唇颊侧牙龈部分还需要烤塑（图28）。

另一方面，切削全瓷外冠、烧结、染色，并粘接至钛桥架的对应位置，在𬌗架上再次调𬌗、抛光，最终完成永久修复体的制作（图29和图30）。

gingival morphology for the permanent restoration. The lingual gingival portion may be appropriately reduced to decrease lingual volume and minimize the patient's sensation of a foreign body. After obtaining the external shape of the permanent restoration, space is created for milling the all-ceramic crowns and the labial and buccal gingival veneers, resulting in the final titanium framework morphology.

Before processing the titanium framework, a PMMA framework can be processed (Fig. 25) to validate the design data and accuracy of the processing equipment. Once everything is verified, the titanium framework can be machined (Fig. 26). Check the positioning of the framework on the dies and the space for crowns. The titanium framework then needs to be shaded (Fig. 27), and the labial and buccal side gingival portion needs to be customized (Fig. 28).

On the other hand, the all-ceramic crowns are milled, sintered, stained, and bonded to the corresponding position on the titanium framework, then adjusted on the framework, polished. And finally, the permanent restoration is completed (Figs. 29 and 30).

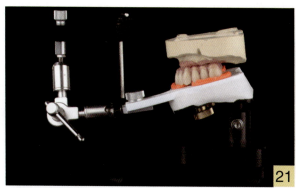

21 上颌模型上𬌗架
Maxillary model set on the articulator

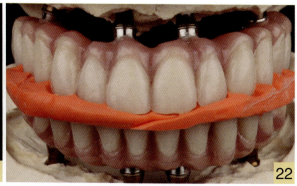

22 下颌模型上𬌗架
Mandibular model set on the articulator

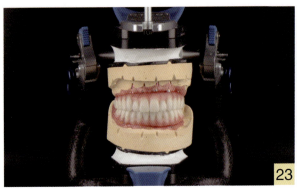

23 评估桥完成
Finished evaluation bridge

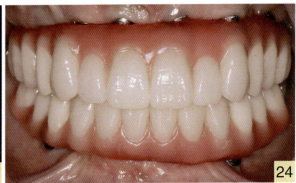

24 试戴评估桥
Try-in of evaluation bridge

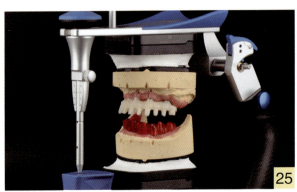

25 PMMA桥架
The PMMA framework

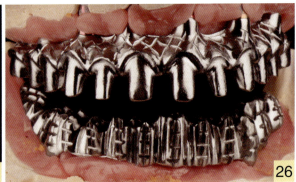

26 钛桥架
The titanium framework

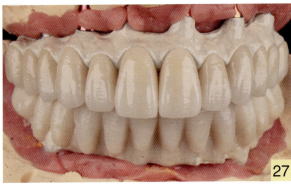

27 钛桥架遮色
Shaded titanium framework

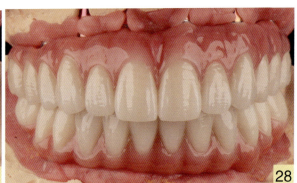

28 钛桥架唇颊侧烤塑
Customized labial and buccal side of gingival portion

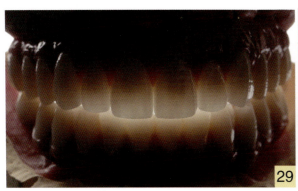

29 透光性良好的冠修复体
Translucent crowns

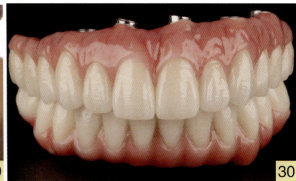

30 完成的永久修复体
Finished definitive restoration

戴牙与随访

被动就位仍然是永久修复体戴牙首要关注的问题，可以拍摄曲面体层片或者根尖片加以确认（图31）。修复体组织面不能压迫牙槽嵴，要有能通过牙缝刷的清洁通道。确定修复体完全就位，且组织面形态合适后，二级螺丝需加力至18Ncm左右，再封闭螺丝孔（图32和图33）。

永久修复体正中咬合接触点也应当广泛、均分地分布，侧方𬌗建议制作为组牙功能𬌗，前伸时多颗前牙均匀引导且后牙不接触。

患者戴牙后1~2周复查口腔卫生维护情况；1个月后再次核查咬合是否正确；之后每半年至一年都需要复诊，检查口腔卫生、咬合是否合适，拍片评估牙槽骨变化等。

Delivery and follow-up

Passive placement is still the primary concern for the permanent restoration of dental implants, which can be confirmed by taking radiographs (Fig. 31). The restoration should not compress the alveolar ridge, and there should be a cleaning channel that interdental brushes can get through. After ensuring that the restoration is completely in place and that the tissue surface morphology is appropriate, the secondary screws should be tightened to about 18Ncm and then the screw holes should be sealed (Figs. 32 and 33).

The contact points should be evenly distributed in central occlusion, and the lateral occlusion should be made as a group function occlusion. In protrusive occlusion, multiple anterior teeth should guide evenly, and the posterior teeth should not contact.

The patient should return for a follow-up on oral hygiene maintenance 1-2 weeks after delivery. Recheck the occlusion after 1 month. Thereafter, follow-up appointments are needed every six months to one year to examine oral hygiene, bite alignment, take X-rays to assess changes in alveolar bone, etc.

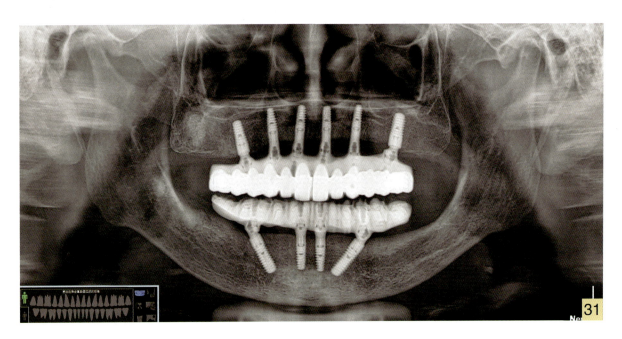

31 戴永久修复体拍摄曲面体层片
Panoramic photography after insertion of the definitive restorations

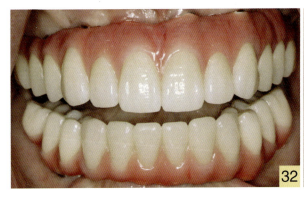

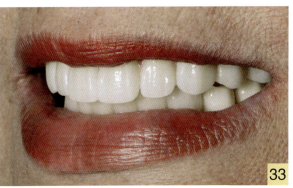

32 戴永久修复体正面小开口照片
Front view of small opening with the definitive restorations

33 戴正式修复体左侧微笑照片
Left view of smile with the definitive restorations

数字化种植修复材料

MATERIALS OF DIGITAL IMPLANT-SUPPORTED RESTORATIONS

第1节　氧化锆多晶陶瓷

Section 1 Multiphase Zirconia

概述及分类

1. 概述

　　氧化锆陶瓷广泛用于制作牙科修复体，主要原因是氧化锆陶瓷具有出色的生物相容性、优异的美学效果和卓越的机械性能。氧化锆陶瓷与口腔组织相容性良好，不易引起过敏或排斥反应，不会对牙龈和周围组织造成损伤或不适。着色后的氧化锆陶瓷外观与自然牙齿相似，能够与周围牙齿无缝融合，提供良好的美观性和口腔舒适感。此外，氧化锆陶瓷还具有高强度、高韧性，能够承受口腔中的咀嚼力，具有良好的耐久性和稳定性，可以长期保持修复体的完整性和功能性。

2. 分类

　　第1代牙科氧化锆多晶陶瓷在3Y-TZP中添加$0.2 \sim 0.5$wt.%Al_2O_3，这种添加剂有以下作用：提高强度，适量的氧化铝能够有效抑制氧化锆晶体的长大，通过细化晶粒提高氧化锆强度；改善稳定性，氧化铝的加入有助于改善氧化锆的晶体结构稳定性，减少其在长期使用过

Overview and classification

1. Overview

Zirconia ceramics are widely used in the production of dental restorations, primarily because they have excellent biocompatibility, outstanding aesthetic effects, and superior mechanical performance. Zirconia ceramics exhibit good compatibility with oral tissues, are less likely to cause allergies or rejection reactions, and do not damage or discomfort the gums and surrounding tissues. Stained zirconia ceramics have a similar appearance to natural teeth, seamlessly blending with surrounding teeth, providing good aesthetics and oral comfort. Additionally, zirconia ceramics also possess high strength and toughness, can withstand chewing forces in the oral cavity, have good durability and stability, and can maintain the integrity and functionality of the restoration for a long time.

2. Classification

The first generation of dental yttria-stabilized zirconia polycrystalline ceramics, which added 0.2-0.5 wt.% Al_2O_3 to 3Y-TZP, serves several functions. The addition of alumina increases strength by effectively inhibiting zirconia crystal growth and refining the grains. It also improves stability by enhancing the crystal structure stability of zirconia, thereby reducing potential aging during long-term use and extending its service life. Furthermore, alumina optimizes other properties of zirconia ceramics, such as the thermal expansion coefficient and chemical stability. This type of zirconia

程中可能出现的老化现象，延长其使用寿命；优化性能，氧化铝的添加还可以优化氧化锆陶瓷的其他性能，如热膨胀系数和化学稳定性，这类氧化锆材料透度不高，更适合用于内冠。

第2代牙科氧化锆多晶陶瓷提升了氧化锆制备工艺，不需要较高Al_2O_3含量也可以提升3Y-TZP的强度和老化性能，这种材料具有以下特点：较低的氧化铝含量，可以在降低氧化铝含量或不加氧化铝的情况下达到1代牙科氧化锆的强度和老化性能；提高透光性，通过降低氧化铝含量，减少了光在晶体内部的散射，2代牙科氧化锆的透光性得到大幅提升，使得材料质感整体提升；新的预染色技术，2代牙科氧化锆采用预染色瓷块逐渐部分取代白色瓷块加染色液方式，这种预染色技术可以在氧化锆制备过程中直接实现所需的颜色，而不需要额外的染色工序，简化了流程，提高了生产效率。

第3代牙科氧化锆多晶陶瓷通过提高稳定剂Y_2O_3含量到5mol%得到5Y-PSZ，这种改进带来了以下优势：大幅提高材料透光性，通过稳定剂Y_2O_3含量的提高，烧结体立方相含量增加，立方相不产生双折射现象，大幅增加了材料的可见光透过率，拓展了氧化锆的适应证范围，可以将这种氧化锆用于前牙或贴面修复；进一步提升老化性能，Y_2O_3含量的提高减少了亚稳定的四方相含量，减少了特殊环境下向单斜相转变的概率，从而提高了材料的老化性能，延长了使用寿命。

第4代牙科氧化锆多晶陶瓷控制稳定剂含量在4mol%，烧结体的微观结构一般含有较多的四方相和少量的立方相，实现了强度和透度

material, characterized by low translucency, is more suitable for use in inner crown.

The second-generation dental zirconia polycrystalline ceramic has improved the preparation process of zirconia, enhancing the strength and aging resistance of 3Y-TZP without the need for high Al_2O_3 content. This material has the following characteristics: lower alumina content, achieving the strength and aging resistance of the first-generation dental zirconia without reducing alumina content or adding alumina; improved translucency by reducing alumina content, reducing light scattering inside the crystal, greatly enhancing the translucency of the second-generation dental zirconia, enhancing the overall texture of the material; and new pre-coloring technology: the second-generation dental zirconia gradually replaces white ceramic blocks with pre-colored ceramic blocks instead of using coloring liquids. This pre-coloring technology can directly achieve the desired color during the preparation of zirconia, without the need for additional coloring processes, simplifying the process and improving production efficiency.

The third generation of dental zirconia polycrystalline ceramics achieved 5Y-PSZ by increasing the Y_2O_3 stabilizer content to 5mol%. This enhancement offers the following benefits: significantly improving the material's light transmittance. By increasing the stabilizer Y_2O_3 content, the amount of cubic phase in the sintered body increases. The cubic phase does not produce birefringence, greatly increasing the visible light transmittance of the material and expanding the indications for zirconia. This allows the zirconia to be used for anterior teeth or veneer restorations, further enhancing the aging performance. The increase in Y_2O_3 content reduces the tetragonal phase content, reducing the probability of transformation to the monoclinic phase in special environments. This improves the material's aging performance and extends its service life.

The 4th generation dental zirconia polycrystalline ceramics control the stabilizer content at 4mol%, and the microstructure of the sintered body generally contains a large amount of tetragonal phase and a small amount of cubic phase, achieving a perfect match between strength and translucency. The strength generally

之间的完美匹配，强度一般可满足全适应证要求，对于长桥修复体透光性也具有一定优势（图1）。

第5代牙科氧化锆多晶陶瓷通过不同Y_2O_3含量粉料的叠加，实现了从切端到颈部透光性和颜色的渐变效果，所谓渐变效果是在制作过程中通过不同瓷层堆叠模拟天然牙色彩层次和透度变化，这种仿生叠层氧化锆材料更加接近天然牙结构，实现了更好的仿真效果，代表了现代牙科修复材料的一个重要进展，它结合了最新的材料科学、数字化技术和美学理念，满足了医生和患者对功能与美学的双重需求（图2）。

此外，还有其他形式的氧化锆材料，全烧结氧化锆是一种椅旁使用的完全烧结的氧化锆瓷块，具有零收缩、免烧结的特点，适合1~3单位的修复体类型，缺点是硬度高，加工成本高。荧光氧化锆是将荧光剂引入到氧化锆陶瓷，在特殊光源的激发下，会发出类似天然牙的蓝白色荧光效果，达到更好的仿真效果。近年来市场上还出了快烧氧化锆、种植桥架专用的氧化锆等。快烧氧化锆在小于1小时的极速烧结条件下仍可以达到预期性能，而种植桥架氧化锆可以满足半口或全口的All-on-4或All-on-6的上部修复，这种材料带有牙龈结构，在实现硬组织修复的同时实现软组织修复（图3）。

meets the requirements of all indications, and also has certain advantages in translucency for long-span restorations(Fig. 1).

The fifth-generation dental zirconia polycrystalline ceramics achieve a gradient effect of translucency and color from the incisal to the cervical by overlapping powders with different Y_2O_3 contents. The so-called gradient effect simulates the natural color layers and translucency changes of teeth through the stacking of different ceramic layers during the manufacturing process. This biomimetic layered zirconia material is closer to the natural tooth structure, achieving a better simulation effect. It represents an important advancement in modern dental restorative materials, combining the latest materials science, digital technology, and aesthetic concepts to meet the dual requirements of functionality and aesthetics for doctors and patients(Fig. 2).

In addition, there are other forms of zirconia materials. Fully sintered zirconia is a fully sintered zirconia ceramic block used chairside, with zero shrinkage and no sintering required, suitable for 1-3 unit restorations. The drawback is its high hardness and processing cost. Fluorescent zirconia introduces a fluorescent agent into zirconia ceramics, which emits a blue-white fluorescence effect similar to natural teeth under special light sources, achieving better aesthetic results. In recent years, there have been advancements in zirconia technology, including fast-sintered zirconia and zirconia specifically designed for implant bridges. Fast-sintered zirconia is able to achieve expected performance even under extreme sintering conditions of less than 1 hour. On the other hand, implant bridge zirconia is capable of meeting the restoration needs for half-mouth or full-mouth All-on-4 or All-on-6 procedures. This material not only simulates the gum structure but also achieves restoration of both hard and soft tissues(Fig. 3).

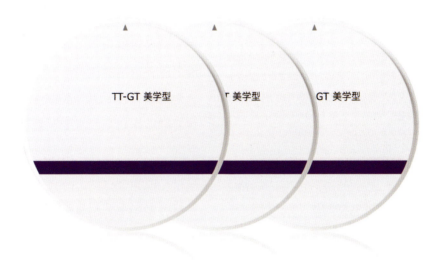

1 用于前牙美学修复的氧化锆
Zirconia for anterior aesthetic restoration

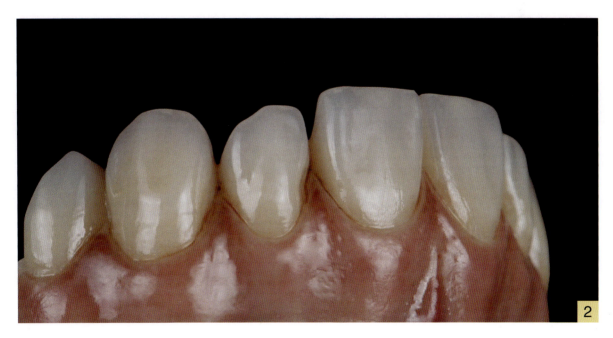

2 具有渐变效果的氧化锆
Zirconia with gradient effect

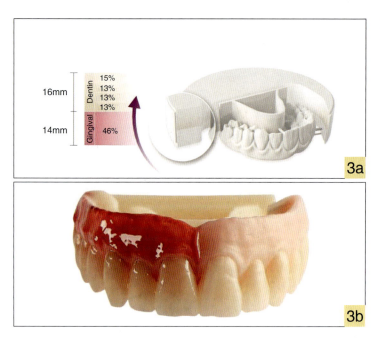

3 全口种植桥架氧化锆
Zirconia framework for full-arch implantation

成分和性能

　　不同代别氧化锆化学成分及性能见表1和表2。

Composition and properties

The chemical composition and properties of different generations of zirconia are shown in Tables 1 and 2, respectively.

表1　不同代别氧化锆化学成分

	1代	2代	3代	4代	5代
Al_2O_3含量（wt.%）	0.2～0.5	低Al_2O_3或无Al_2O_3	低Al_2O_3或无Al_2O_3	低Al_2O_3或无Al_2O_3	低Al_2O_3或无Al_2O_3
Y_2O_3含量（mol%）	3	3	5	4	3～5或3～4或4～5
Eu_2O_3（wt.%）	< 0.4	< 0.4	< 0.4	< 0.4	< 0.4
Fe_2O_3（wt.%）	< 0.1	< 0.1	< 0.1	< 0.1	< 0.1
Mn_2O_3（wt.%）	< 0.0004	< 0.0004	< 0.0004	< 0.0004	< 0.0004
Nd_2O_3（wt.%）	< 0.0004	< 0.0004	< 0.0004	< 0.0004	< 0.0004

Table 1 Chemical composition of different generations of zirconia

	1st	2nd	3rd	4th	5th
Al_2O_3 content (wt.%)	0.2-0.5	Low Al_2O_3 or no Al_2O_3	Low Al_2O_3 or no Al_2O_3	Low Al_2O_3 or no Al_2O_3	Low Al_2O_3 or no Al_2O_3
Y_2O_3 content (mol%)	3	3	5	4	3-5 or 3-4 or 4-5
Eu_2O_3 (wt.%)	< 0.4	< 0.4	< 0.4	< 0.4	< 0.4
Fe_2O_3 (wt.%)	< 0.1	< 0.1	< 0.1	< 0.1	< 0.1
Mn_2O_3 (wt.%)	< 0.0004	< 0.0004	< 0.0004	< 0.0004	< 0.0004
Nd_2O_3 (wt.%)	< 0.0004	< 0.0004	< 0.0004	< 0.0004	< 0.0004

表2 不同代别氧化锆性能

	1代	2代	3代	4代	5代
Y_2O_3含量（mol%）	3	3	5	4	3~5
三点弯曲强度（MPa）	1100~1300	1100~1300	600~700	900~1000	600~1300
维氏硬度（GPa）	12~13	12~13	12~13	12~13	12~13
弹性模量（GPa）	190~220	190~220	190~220	190~220	190~220
可见光透过率（%）	39	43	49	46	43~46
热膨胀系数（10^{-6}/K）	10.5±0.5	10.5±0.5	10.5±0.5	10.5±0.5	10.5±0.5

Table 2 Performance of different generations of zirconia

	1st	2nd	3rd	4th	5th
Y_2O_3 content (mol%)	3	3	5	4	3-5
Three-point flexural strength (MPa)	1100-1300	1100-1300	600-700	900-1000	600-1300
Vickers hardness (GPa)	12-13	12-13	12-13	12-13	12-13
Elastic modulus (GPa)	190-220	190-220	190-220	190-220	190-220
Visible light transmittance (%)	39	43	49	46	43-46
Thermal expansion coefficient (10^{-6}/K)	10.5±0.5	10.5±0.5	10.5±0.5	10.5±0.5	10.5±0.5

优缺点

氧化锆陶瓷作为牙科修复材料具有许多优点，但也有一些局限性，以下是其主要的优缺点：

1. 优点

生物相容性良好：氧化锆陶瓷与口腔组织相容性高，不易引起过敏或排斥反应，能够长期稳定地与周围组织相处。

优异的美学效果：高透氧化锆着色后的外观与自然牙齿相似度高，能够提供良好的美观性和口腔舒适感。

Advantages and disadvantages

Zirconia ceramic as a dental restoration material has many advantages, but also has some limitations. The following are its main pros and cons:

1. Advantages

Good biocompatibility: Zirconia ceramics have high compatibility with oral tissues, are less likely to cause allergic or rejection reactions, and can stably coexist with surrounding tissues for an extended period.

Excellent aesthetic effects: The appearance of high-translucent zirconia after coloring is highly similar to natural teeth, providing good aesthetics and oral comfort.

高强度：氧化锆陶瓷具有优异的挠曲强度，能够承受口腔中的咀嚼力，具有良好的耐久性和稳定性。

抗氧化性：氧化锆陶瓷具有良好的抗氧化性，能够长期保持其原有的颜色和外观，不易发生氧化或褪色。

2. 缺点

脆性：尽管氧化锆陶瓷具有高强度，但在极端情况下仍可能发生破裂或断裂，尤其是在应力集中的区域。

导热性较差：相较于金属材料，氧化锆陶瓷的导热性较差，可能导致修复体与周围牙齿之间的温度差异，引起不适感或牙髓刺激。

低温老化现象：口腔湿热环境可能会导致 Y_2O_3 析出，导致四方相向单斜相的转变，引起强度的下降。

氧化锆硬度远高于天然牙，会对对颌牙造成磨损，但是高度抛光后磨损明显减少，综合来看，尽管氧化锆陶瓷具有许多优点，但在选择牙科修复材料时，仍需要综合考虑患者的口腔状况、修复需求以及经济能力等因素，以确定最适合的修复方案。

临床应用

根据ISO6872/GB30367，当烧结后的氧化锆瓷块的挠曲强度在300~500MPa时，可用于制作贴面、嵌体、单冠及不包含磨牙的3单位修复体的基底陶瓷；当烧结后的牙科用氧化锆瓷块的挠曲强度大于500MPa时，可用于制作贴面、

High strength: Zirconia ceramics have excellent flexural strength, can withstand the chewing forces in the oral cavity, and exhibit good durability and stability.

Antioxidant property: Zirconia ceramics have excellent antioxidant property, which can maintain their original color and appearance for a long time without oxidation or discoloration.

2. Disadvantages

Brittleness: Although zirconia ceramics have high strength, they may still experience cracking or fracture under extreme conditions, especially in areas of stress concentration.

Poor thermal conductivity is a characteristic of zirconia ceramic when compared to metal materials. This difference in thermal conductivity may result in temperature variations between the restoration and the surrounding teeth, potentially causing discomfort or pulpal stimulation.

Low-temperature aging phenomenon occurs in the oral moist and hot environment. This may lead to the precipitation of Y_2O_3, causing the transformation from tetragonal phase to monoclinic phase, resulting in a decrease in strength.

The hardness of zirconia is significantly higher than that of natural teeth, which can lead to wear on opposing teeth. However, this wear can be greatly reduced through high-level polishing. Overall, although zirconia ceramics have many advantages, when choosing dental restorative materials, it is still necessary to consider factors such as the patient's oral condition, restoration needs, and economic capabilities to determine the most suitable restorative solution.

Clinical application

According to ISO6872/GB30367, when the flexural strength of sintered zirconia ceramic blocks is between 300-500MPa, they can be used as the substructure ceramic material for veneers, inlays, single crowns, and three-unit restorations without molar grinding. When the flexural strength of sintered dental zirconia ceramic blocks is greater than 500MPa, they can be used as the substructure ceramic material for veneers, inlays, single

嵌体、单冠及包含磨牙的3单位修复体的基底陶瓷；当烧结后的牙科用氧化锆瓷块的挠曲强度大于800MPa时，可用于制作贴面、嵌体、单冠及包含4单位及以上修复体的基底陶瓷。氧化锆多晶陶瓷定位为冠桥材料，具有较宽的适应证需求。详见表3。

应用指导

1. 设计加工

数字化扫描：首先对需要修复的牙齿或牙模进行数字化扫描，以获取口腔结构的精确三维模型数据。可以通过口腔内部的激光扫描仪或外部的牙模扫描仪来实现。

crowns, and three-unit restorations including molars. When the flexural strength of sintered dental zirconia ceramic blocks is greater than 800MPa, they can be used as the substructure ceramic material for veneers, inlays, single crowns, and four-unit or more restorations, with zirconia polycrystalline ceramics positioned as crown and bridge materials, meeting a wide range of clinical needs. See Table 3 for details.

Application guidance

1. Design and processing

Digital scanning: First, a digital scan is taken of the teeth or dental models that need to be repaired to obtain precise three-dimensional model data of the oral structure. This can be achieved through an intraoral laser scanner or an external dental model scanner.

表3 不同代别氧化锆适应证

适应证	1代	2代	3代	4代	5代	
					3Y-4Y	4Y-5Y
内冠	++	+	+	+	+	+
嵌体/高嵌体/贴面	+	+	+	+	+	+
全解剖形态/结构的前牙/后牙冠	+	+	++	+	+	++
最多3单位的全解剖形态/结构的前牙桥（不超过一个缺失位）*	+	+	++	++	+	++
全解剖形态/结构的多单位前牙桥（大于等于4单位，不超过两个连续的缺失位）*	+	+	−	++	++	−
种植上部的半口/全口长桥修复*	+	+	−	−	++	−

++ 强烈推荐；+ 可用于此适应证；− 未指明

*基于固定修复的设计原则

Table 3 Indications for Different Generations of Zirconia

Adaptation Criteria	Generation 1	Generation 2	Generation 3	Generation 4	Generation 5	
					3Y-4Y	4Y-5Y
Inner crowns	++	+	+	+	+	+
Inlays/Onlays/Veneers	+	+	+	+	+	+
Full anatomical form/ structure of anterior/ posterior crowns	+	+	++	+	+	++
Up to 3-unit full anatomical form/structure anterior bridge (no more than one missing unit)*	+	+	++	++	+	++
More than 4-unit full anatomical form/structure anterior bridge (greater than or equal to 4 units, no more than two consecutive missing units)*	+	+	–	++	++	–
Implant support of half/ full upper long bridge restoration*	+	+	–	–	++	–

++ Highly recommended, + Applicable for this indication, - Not specified
*Based on the principle of fixed repairs

计算机辅助设计（CAD）：使用CAD软件，将扫描得到的口腔模型数据导入计算机中，进行修复体的数字化设计。在CAD软件中，牙科技师可以根据患者的具体情况，设计出符合口腔解剖结构和修复需求的氧化锆修复体。

数控加工（CAM）：设计完成后，将修复体的CAD数据导入数控加工设备中进行加工，将氧化锆陶瓷块精确加工成所需形态的修复体。

Computer-aided design (CAD): Using CAD software, the scanned oral model data is imported into the computer for digital design of the restoration. In the CAD software, dental technicians can design zirconia restorations that meet the specific oral anatomical structure and restoration needs of the patient.

Computer-aided manufacturing (CAM): After the design is completed, the CAD data of the restoration is imported into the CAM system for precise processing of the zirconia ceramic block into the desired form of the restoration.

2. 染色

氧化锆坯体的染色方式一般有两种：浸泡和涂刷，浸泡一般将修复体完全浸入到一定浓度的染色液中，根据染色液具体要求设定浸泡时间，完成浸泡后去除多余液体，然后充分干燥；涂刷一般使用细小的毛刷在修复体表面涂上一层薄薄的染色液，可分多次涂刷以构建出自然的色泽层次和渐变效果，最后充分干燥。

对于预着色瓷块，一般可以无需染色直接烧结，有时为了增加切端效果，也可以在切端涂刷增透染色液。

3. 烧结

氧化锆陶瓷的烧结过程是将坯体在高温下进行热处理，以实现颗粒之间的结合和致密化，达到其理论密度从而发挥最终性能。牙科氧化锆烧结温度一般为1450℃～1550℃，最高温度保温时间10～180分钟，按烧结总时间我们可以将牙科氧化锆的烧结分为几类，总时间8～10小时的常规烧结、总时间4小时左右的技工间快烧、总时间2小时左右的临床快烧和1小时以内的极速烧结。烧结炉按加热方式一般可分为硅钼棒烧结炉、硅碳棒烧结炉、感应加热烧结炉、微波加热烧结炉以及低真空烧结炉等。烧结制度会对材料的强度、透度、颜色等产生影响，为了达到最佳的机械和光学性能，需要遵守规定的烧结温度和时间。

2. Dyeing

The dyeing of zirconia blanks is generally done in two ways: brushing and immersion. Immersion involves fully immersing the restoration in a dye solution of a certain concentration, setting the immersion time according to the specific requirements of the dye solution, removing excess liquid after immersion, and allowing it to dry thoroughly. Brushing typically involves using a fine brush to apply a thin layer of dye solution to the surface of the restoration, which can be applied multiple times to create natural color layers and gradient effects, followed by thorough drying.

Pre-colored blocks can generally be sintered without the need for dyeing. Sometimes, for the purpose of enhancing the incisal effect, a translucency enhancing dye can also be applied to the incisal.

3. Sintering

The sintering process of zirconia ceramics involves heat treating the green body at high temperatures to achieve particle bonding and densification, reaching its theoretical density for the final performance. The sintering temperature for dental zirconia is generally between 1450-1550°C, with a holding time of 10-180 minutes at the highest temperature. Based on the total sintering time, dental zirconia sintering can be classified into several categories: conventional sintering with a total time of 8-10 hours, technician quick sintering with a total time of around 4 hours, clinical quick sintering with a total time of around 2 hours, and ultra-fast sintering within 1 hour. Sintering furnaces can be divided into types such as silicon molybdenum rod sintering furnace, silicon carbide rod sintering furnace, induction heating sintering furnace, microwave heating sintering furnace, and low vacuum sintering furnace based on heating methods. The sintering process will affect the material's strength, translucency, color, etc. To achieve the best mechanical and optical performance, it is necessary to adhere to the specified sintering temperature and time.

4. 打磨、抛光

氧化锆陶瓷的打磨抛光是指通过机械或化学方法，对氧化锆陶瓷表面进行加工，以获得光滑、亮泽且无瑕疵的表面质感。

粗磨：在初始阶段，使用颗粒较大的磨料对氧化锆陶瓷表面进行粗磨。这一步旨在降低表面的粗糙度、减少表面缺陷，并初步塑造所需的形状。

细磨：经过粗磨后，采用颗粒较小的磨料对氧化锆陶瓷表面进行细磨，进一步平整表面、减少磨痕和提高表面光滑度。对于5Y-PSZ产品，由于强度和韧性相对较低，打磨工具及参数可参考玻璃陶瓷产品。

抛光：经过细磨后，使用抛光工艺对氧化锆陶瓷表面进行抛光处理。抛光可以利用高速旋转的抛光轮或抛光液等，使表面获得更高的光泽度，进一步减少微小的瑕疵和磨痕。

清洁和检查：完成抛光后，对氧化锆陶瓷进行清洁，以去除表面残留的磨料和抛光液等。随后进行表面检查，确保表面质量符合要求。在整个打磨抛光过程中，需要严格控制加工参数，如磨料选择、压力、速度和时间等，以确保获得一致的表面质量和光泽度。

5. 外染

氧化锆陶瓷的外染是指在氧化锆陶瓷表面施加染色剂或采用特定的染色工艺，以改变其表面颜色或实现特定的视觉效果，有助于使氧化锆陶瓷修复体看起来更加自然，并与患者的其他牙齿协调一致（图4）。

4. Grinding and polishing

The grinding and polishing of zirconia ceramics refers to the processing of the surface of zirconia ceramics through mechanical or chemical methods to obtain a smooth, glossy, and flawless surface texture.

Rough grinding: In the initial stage, use larger abrasive particles to rough grind the surface of zirconia ceramics. This step aims to reduce surface roughness, decrease surface defects, and preliminarily shape the desired form.

Polishing: After rough grinding, use abrasives with smaller particles to fine-grind the surface of zirconia ceramics, further smoothing the surface, reducing scratches, and improving surface smoothness. For 5Y-PSZ products, due to their relatively lower strength and toughness, polishing tools and parameters can refer to glass ceramic products.

Polishing: After fine grinding, the surface of zirconia ceramic is polished using polishing techniques. Polishing can be done using high-speed rotating polishing wheels or polishing liquids to achieve a higher gloss on the surface, further reducing minor flaws and scratches.

Cleaning and Inspection: After polishing, it is important to clean the zirconia ceramics to remove any residual abrasives and polishing compounds on the surface. This step is crucial in ensuring the final product meets quality standards. Following the cleaning process, a thorough surface inspection should be conducted to verify that the surface quality meets the specified requirements. Throughout the grinding and polishing process, it is necessary to strictly control processing parameters such as abrasive selection, pressure, speed, and time to ensure consistent surface quality and glossiness.

5. Glazing and staining

Zirconia ceramic external staining refers to applying a coloring agent on the surface of zirconia ceramics or using specific coloring techniques to change its surface color or achieve specific visual effects, which helps make zirconia ceramic restorations look more natural and harmonize with the patient's other teeth(Fig. 4).

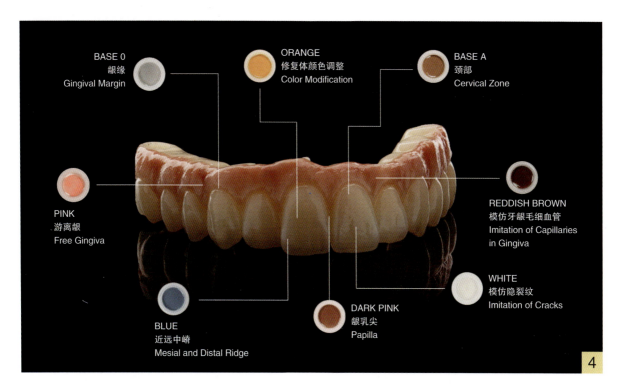

4 常见外染釉膏的颜色体系和应用指导
Provides a color system and application guide for common external glazed and stained color. The guide helps users understand how to effectively use different colors in their external glazing and staining projects

6. 粘接

　　评价修复成功的标准不仅需要修复体满足优异的力学性能、生物相容性和化学稳定性，还需要修复体与牙体之间形成稳固的粘接力。修复体的表面处理主要有两类，一种是表面粗糙化，清除修复体表面污染物并改善表面微结构，使其能与粘接剂形成良好的微机械锁结，满足机械固位。常用的方法有打磨、喷砂、氢氟酸蚀刻及激光等。另一种方法是表面改性，改变修复体表面化学性质，增强修复体与粘接剂之间的亲和力，从而获得增加粘接力的效果。

6. Adhesion

The evaluation criteria for successful restoration not only require the restorative material to meet excellent mechanical properties, biocompatibility, and chemical stability but also require a strong bond to be formed between the restoration and the tooth structure. There are mainly two types of surface treatments for restorative materials. One method is surface roughening, which involves removing surface contaminants and improving the surface microstructure to allow for a good micromechanical lock with the adhesive, meeting the mechanical retention requirements. Common methods include polishing, sandblasting, hydrofluoric acid etching, and laser treatment. The other method is surface modification, which involves altering the chemical properties of the restorative material surface to enhance the affinity between the restorative material and the adhesive, thereby increasing the bonding strength.

喷砂是临床应用较广泛的常规技术，喷砂可使氧化锆陶瓷表面粗糙，产生不规则的表面，以增加粘接表面的表面积，提高单位面积的粘接强度并有效消除表面污染，提供表面清洁。因为缺乏玻璃相晶体，氧化锆陶瓷在常温下、短时间内几乎不会被氢氟酸酸蚀，酸蚀效果不佳。除非使用较高浓度氢氟酸、延长酸蚀时间或者提高温度，如高浓度氢氟酸（>40%）在加热（100℃）下，并延长酸蚀时间（30分钟至2小时）对氧化锆表面有一定的酸蚀作用。

磷酸酯单体已被证明能与氧化锆形成化学结合，常用的可聚合的有机磷酸酯单体是MDP，它通过一端的磷酸基团，能够与氧化锆陶瓷表面的金属氧化物水合层形成氢键、离子键或者配位键，而单体另一端的双键可以与甲基丙烯酸树脂共聚合，从而显著提高树脂与氧化锆陶瓷的粘接强度。现阶段常用的通用型粘接剂和氧化锆专用处理剂中均含有MDP成分。

氧化锆陶瓷表面缺少玻璃相，传统的硅烷偶联剂并不适用于氧化锆陶瓷的表面处理，可用摩擦化学的方法在氧化锆陶瓷表面黏附一层二氧化硅涂层，再用硅烷偶联剂处理。

Sandblasting is a widely used conventional technique in clinical applications. Sandblasting can roughen the surface of zirconia ceramic, creating an irregular surface to increase the bonding surface area, improve the bonding strength per unit area, effectively eliminate surface contamination, and provide surface cleanliness. Due to the lack of glass-phase crystals, zirconia ceramics are hardly corroded by hydrofluoric acid at room temperature and for a short period of time, leading to poor acid etching effects. Only when using higher concentrations of hydrofluoric acid, extending the etching time, or raising the temperature, such as higher concentrations of hydrofluoric acid (>40%) at a heating temperature of 100°C, and prolonging the etching time (30 minutes to 2 hours), can there be a certain etching effect on the surface of zirconia.

Phosphate ester monomers, such as MDP, have been found to chemically bond with zirconia. These monomers can form various types of bonds with the metal oxide hydroxide layer on the zirconia ceramic surface, including hydrogen bonds, ionic bonds, and coordination bonds. The phosphate group on one end of the monomer interacts with the ceramic surface, while the double bond on the other end can copolymerize with the methacrylate resin. This interaction significantly enhances the bonding strength between the resin and the zirconia ceramic. Both universal adhesives and zirconia-specific primers currently used contain MDP component.

The surface of zirconia ceramics lacks a glass phase. Traditional silane coupling agents are not suitable for surface treatment of zirconia ceramics. A layer of silicon dioxide coating can be adhered to the surface of zirconia ceramics by frictional chemical method, and then treated with silane coupling agents.

第2节 牙科玻璃基陶瓷

Section 2 Dental Glass–based Ceramics

概述及分类

玻璃基陶瓷是一种具有玻璃和陶瓷双重特性的材料，通常由氧化硅、氧化铝、氧化锂等成分组成。它具有优异的耐高温性、化学稳定性和机械性能，同时还具有类似于玻璃的透明度和光泽度，通常用于牙科美学修复。

1. 玻璃基陶瓷分类（按应用）

（1）热压铸玻璃陶瓷。热压铸玻璃陶瓷简称铸瓷，它是将玻璃陶瓷在高温、高压下注入型腔并烧结、制作全瓷修复体的陶瓷。热压铸方法有助于避免瓷体中形成大空隙，提高了材料致密度和强度，可促使玻璃陶瓷基质中晶粒定向排列，可以得到较高的强度。瓷修复体的收缩可通过包埋料的热膨胀加以补偿，故其边缘适合性好。同时半透明性优异，常用于超薄贴面。

（2）可加工玻璃陶瓷。可加工玻璃陶瓷是指利用现代数字化技术设计并加工制造的玻璃基陶瓷修复材料。

Overview and classification

Glass-based ceramics are materials with dual properties of glass and ceramics, usually composed of components such as silica, alumina, and lithium oxide. They exhibit excellent high temperature resistance, chemical stability, and mechanical performance, as well as transparency and luster similar to glass, and are commonly used in aesthetic dental restorations.

1. Classification of glass-ceramics (by application)

(1) Hot-pressed glass ceramics. Hot-pressed glass ceramics, known as cast ceramics, is the process of injecting glass ceramics into a mold cavity at high temperature and pressure, and sintering to produce an all-ceramic restoration. The hot-pressing method helps to avoid the formation of large voids in the ceramic body, increases the material density and strength, and can promote the oriented arrangement of grains in the glass ceramic matrix to achieve higher strength. The shrinkage of the ceramic restoration can be compensated by the thermal expansion of the embedding material, resulting in good marginal fit. It also has excellent translucency and is commonly used for ultra-thin veneers.

(2) CAD/CAM glass ceramics. Glass-ceramics for restoration materials are those designed and processed using modern digital technologies.

2. 玻璃基陶瓷分类（按成分）

（1）长石。这种材料通常包含长石（一种含有钾钠钙的天然矿物）为主要成分，采用浇铸法或烧结法制备而成，具有一定半透性，强度较低，适合前牙美学区修复。

（2）白榴石。白榴石增强微晶玻璃（$SiO_2-Al_2O_3-K_2O$体系）是玻璃基体中含有45%左右体积分数的四方白榴石（$KAlSi_2O_6$）晶体的一类微晶玻璃。白榴石晶体的折射率（1.508）与白榴石基质玻璃的折射率（1.47~1.51）比较接近，使得白榴石微晶玻璃的透光率高于其他材料，具有极佳的美学性能。

（3）二硅酸锂增强型玻璃陶瓷。二硅酸锂玻璃陶瓷（$Li_2Si_2O_5$）是一种被广泛应用于口腔修复的材料，力学性能得到了较大突破，强度和韧性均明显提高，主要原因是产生了机械互锁的微观结构，适应证也得到了扩展，可用于前牙3单位桥。

（4）锆增强型二硅酸锂。此类材料试图通过加入锆颗粒或锆氧化合物，来提高材料的弯曲强度和韧性，但实际并未取得预期效果，反而制备工艺相对复杂。

表4和表5分别列出了玻璃陶瓷化学成分和性能。

2. Classification of glass-based ceramics (by composition)

(1) Feldspathic porcelain, typically consisting of feldspar (a natural mineral containing potassium, sodium, and calcium) as the main component, is prepared by casting or sintering. It has a certain degree of translucency and low strength, making it suitable for aesthetic restorations in the anterior dental region.

(2) Leucite, a type of microcrystalline glass in the $SiO_2-Al_2O_3-K_2O$ system, contains about 45% volume fraction of leucite ($KAlSi_2O_6$) crystals in the glass matrix. The refractive index of leucite crystal (1.508) is close to that of the leucite matrix (1.47-1.51), resulting in higher light transmission of leucite compared to other materials. This glass also boasts excellent aesthetic properties.

(3) Enhanced lithium disilicate glass ceramics. Lithium disilicate glass ceramics ($Li_2Si_2O_5$) are materials widely used in dental restoration. They have shown significant improvements in mechanical properties, including increased strength and toughness. The main reason for these improvements is the development of a microstructure with mechanical interlocks. The indications have also been expanded, and it can be used for a 3-unit anterior bridge.

(4) Zirconia enhanced lithium disilicate. It is a type of material that aims to enhance bending strength and toughness by incorporating zirconia particles or zirconium compounds. However, the actual results did not meet expectations, and instead, the preparation process became relatively complex.

Chemical composition and properties of glass ceramics are in Tables 4 and 5.

表4　玻璃陶瓷化学成分

成分	长石	白榴石	二硅酸锂	锆增强型二硅酸锂
SiO_2	56 ~ 64	59 ~ 63	58 ~ 72.5	49 ~ 72.5
Al_2O_3	19 ~ 25	19 ~ 25	0 ~ 4	0 ~ 4
Li_2O	—	—	10 ~ 15	10 ~ 25
K_2O	6 ~ 8	10 ~ 14	0.1 ~ 5	0.1 ~ 5
Na_2O	6 ~ 9	3.5 ~ 6.5	0 ~ 4	0 ~ 4
ZrO_2	—	—	0 ~ 3	8 ~ 20

Table 4 Chemical Composition of Glass Ceramics

Component	Feldspar	Leucite	Lithium Disilicate	Zirconia Enhanced Lithium Disilicate
SiO_2	56-64	59-63	58-72.5	49-72.5
Al_2O_3	19-25	19-25	0-4	0-4
Li_2O	—	—	10-15	10-25
K_2O	6-8	10-14	0.1-5	0.1-5
Na_2O	6-9	3.5-6.5	0-4	0-4
ZrO_2	—	—	0-3	8-20

表5　玻璃陶瓷性能

	长石	白榴石	二硅酸锂	锆增强型二硅酸锂
双轴弯曲强度（MPa）	100 ~ 160	120 ~ 180	300 ~ 420	200 ~ 260
弹性模量（GPa）	45 ~ 65	45 ~ 65	70 ~ 110	70 ~ 110

Table 5 Properties of glass ceramics

	Feldspar	Leucite	Lithium Disilicate	Zirconia Enhanced Lithium Disilicate
Biaxial flexural strength (MPa)	100-160	120-180	300-420	200-260
Young's modulus (GPa)	45-65	45-65	70-110	70-110

优缺点

1. 优点

由于玻璃相的存在，透光性较好，质感更接近天然牙，可实现超薄贴面微创修复，同时可酸蚀硅烷处理，粘接效果良好。

Advantages and disadvantages

1. Advantages

Due to the presence of glass phase, it has good light transmission, a texture closer to natural teeth, and allows for ultra-thin veneer minimally invasive restorations. It can also undergo silane treatment for good adhesive effect.

2. 缺点

强度和韧性没有氧化锆高，不适合长桥修复。

临床应用

嵌体、高嵌体、贴面、超薄贴面、单冠、前牙三联桥（强度大于300MPa）。

应用指导

1. CAD工艺流程

（1）设计加工

数字化扫描：首先对需要修复的牙齿或牙模进行数字化扫描，以获取口腔结构的精确三维模型数据。

计算机辅助设计（CAD）：使用CAD软件，将扫描得到的口腔模型数据导入计算机中，进行修复体的数字化设计。在CAD软件中，牙科技师可以根据患者的具体情况，设计出符合口腔解剖结构和修复需求的玻璃陶瓷修复体。

数控加工（CAM）：设计完成后，将修复体的CAD数据导入数控加工设备中进行加工。数控加工设备根据CAD设计数据，自动控制工具的移动和加工过程，将玻璃陶瓷块精确加工成所需形态的修复体。

（2）打磨抛光

打磨：打磨修复体与连接杆连接部分，使玻璃陶瓷边缘光滑并且没有锐利的边角。

2. Disadvantages

The strength and toughness of this material are not as high as that of zirconia, making it unsuitable for long bridge restorations.

Clinical applications

Inlays, onlays, veneers, ultra-thin veneers, single crowns, and anterior three-unit bridges (with a strength greater than 300MPa).

Application guide

1. CAD process flow

(1) Design for manufacturing

Digital scanning: Firstly, a digital scan is performed on the teeth or dental models that need to be repaired to obtain accurate three-dimensional model data of the oral structure.

Computer-Aided Design (CAD): Using CAD software, the scanned oral model data is imported into the computer for the digital design of restorations. In CAD software, dental technicians can design glass ceramic restorations that meet the oral anatomical structure and restoration needs of patients based on their specific conditions.

CAM (Computer-Aided Manufacturing): After the design is completed, the CAD data of the restoration is imported into the CAM equipment for processing. The CAM equipment automatically controls the movement of the tools and the processing process based on the CAD design data, accurately processing the glass ceramic block into the desired shape of the restoration.

(2) Polishing and buffing

Polishing: Polish and repair the connection between the polishing compound and the connecting rod to make the glass ceramic edges smooth and free of sharp corners.

抛光：在需要的情况下，可以对玻璃陶瓷进行抛光，以增强其表面的光泽度和质感，减少表面缺陷。

（3）晶化上釉

晶化处理：是指将修复体放置在适当的温度下，使其内部结构发生晶化反应的过程，这有助于增强修复体的硬度和稳定性。晶化处理的温度和时间需要根据修复体材料的特性和设计要求进行调整。

上釉：上釉是为了增强修复体表面的光泽度和美观度，上釉可以在晶化处理后进行，通常采用涂覆或喷涂的方式将适当的釉料施加到修复体表面，然后经过烘干或烧结使其固化。对于玻璃陶瓷来说，晶化和上釉有时可以同时完成（图5）。

2. 热压铸工艺流程

热压铸采用失蜡法（lost−wax）制作修复体：蜡型用磷酸盐包埋料包埋，预烧，设定热

Polishing: If necessary, glass ceramics can be polished to enhance the surface gloss and texture, and reduce surface defects.

(3) Glazing and Crystallization

Crystallization treatment: Refers to the process of placing the restoration at the appropriate temperature to induce a crystallization reaction within its internal structure, which helps enhance the hardness and stability of the restoration. The temperature and time of crystallization treatment need to be adjusted according to the characteristics of the restoration material and design requirements.

Glazing is used to enhance the gloss and aesthetics of the surface of the restoration. It is typically done after a crystallization treatment, where an appropriate glaze is applied to the surface of the restoration through coating or spraying, and then cured through drying or firing. For glass ceramics, crystallization and glazing can sometimes be completed simultaneously(Fig. 5).

2. Heat pressed

The lost-wax method is used in hot-pressing casting to produce restorations. The process involves embedding the wax pattern in phosphate investment, pre-firing it, setting hot-press casting parameters, and injecting viscous glass ceramic material into the wax pattern cavity at a specific hot-pressing temperature and pressure. This

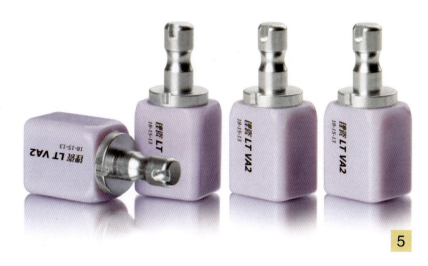

5　二硅酸锂增强型玻璃陶瓷
　　Lithium disilicate-reinforced glass-ceramic

压铸参数，在特定的热压温度下将黏滞的玻璃陶瓷材料以一定的压力注入蜡型空腔，完成瓷修复体的制备，具体步骤如下：

（1）蜡型准备。将修复体的CAD数据导入数控加工设备中加工出蜡型。

（2）铸道安插。铸道始终要沿陶瓷材料流动的方向，安插在蜡型制作的最厚部位，以免影响铸瓷材料的流动性。根据包埋体的数量，选择适当的包埋圈系统。铸造之前，称量包埋圈底座并记录重量。

（3）包埋。浇注包埋料时，要沿着铸圈的边缘缓慢倾倒，可以有效地防止蜡道的脱落和减少气泡的产生，同时振荡机要以最低的振荡能级，包埋充填铸模。

（4）预热（烧圈）。包埋圈按照包埋材料规定的时间固化后，旋去硅橡胶胶圈顶盖和底座，小心把包埋圈自硅橡胶圈中推出，用刮刀平整包埋圈底部表面的粗糙，把包埋圈铸口向下放入预热炉中预热。

（5）压铸。将冷铸瓷块放入热的包埋圈中，将冷的氧化铝推杆涂上分离剂后，放入包埋圈，将包埋圈放入热的铸瓷炉中央，按开始按钮启动所选择的压铸程序。

（6）去包埋。在冷的铸圈上标记氧化铝推杆的长度，用分离盘切割包埋圈。分离推杆和陶瓷材料，用石膏刀在预定的破裂点分离铸圈，用4bar（60psi）的压力进行粗喷砂，用2bar（30psi）的压力进行细喷砂。

（7）其他步骤同CAD工艺。

completes the preparation of the ceramic restoration. The specific steps are as follows:

(1) Wax pattern preparation. Import the CAD data of the repair body into the CNC machining equipment to machine the wax pattern.

(2) Casting channel placement. The casting channel should always follow the direction of the flow of the ceramic material, and be placed at the thickest part of the wax pattern to avoid affecting the flowability of the casting material. Depending on the number of embedded units, choose the appropriate embedding ring system. Before casting, weigh the embedding ring base and record the weight.

(3) Investing. When pouring the embedding material, pour it slowly along the edge of the casting ring. This can effectively prevent the wax pattern from falling off and reduce the generation of air bubbles. At the same time, the vibrating machine should use the lowest vibration energy level to embed and fill the mold.

(4) Preheating (Burnout phase). After curing the embedding ring for the specified time according to the embedding material, remove the silicone rubber ring cover and base, carefully push the embedding ring out from the silicone rubber ring, use a scraper to smooth the rough surface of the bottom of the embedding ring, and place the casting sprue down into the preheating furnace for preheating.

(5) Die casting. Place the cold-pressed block into a hot investment ring, coat the cold alumina push rod with a release agent, place it into the investment ring, position the investment ring in the center of the hot casting furnace, and initiate the selected die casting program by pressing the start button.

(6) Removing investment. Mark the length of the alumina rod on the cold investment ring, cut the embedding ring with a separating disc, and then carefully place the rod into the investment material before allowing it to set. Separate the rod and ceramic material, divide the investment ring at the predetermined break point with a gypsum knife, rough blast with 4 bar (60psi) pressure, and fine blast with 2 bar (30psi) pressure.

(7) The other steps are the same as those in the CAD process.

3. 粘接

对玻璃陶瓷而言，氢氟酸是酸蚀效果最好的酸蚀剂，氢氟酸（HF）与玻璃陶瓷表面的二氧化硅反应而溶解二氧化硅：

$$4HF + SiO_2 = SiF_4 \uparrow + 2H_2O$$

由于玻璃陶瓷结构中的晶相和玻璃相耐酸蚀能力不同，玻璃相更容易被酸蚀，所以玻璃陶瓷经氢氟酸酸蚀后，表面形成凹凸不平的蜂窝状结构，利于机械固位。酸蚀后需用大量水冲洗，最好超声清洗，以彻底去除附着于瓷表面的氢氟酸与瓷的反应产物。

氢氟酸酸蚀后的玻璃陶瓷表面富含Si-OH，它容易与硅烷偶联剂［如3-甲基丙烯酰氧基丙基三甲氧基硅烷（MPS）］发生化学反应形成-Si-O-化学键。而硅烷偶联剂的另一端的甲基丙烯酸酯键又可以与丙烯酸树脂类粘接剂聚合，最终使粘接剂与玻璃陶瓷形成化学性粘接（图6）。

3. Adhesion

For glass ceramics, hydrofluoric acid is the most effective etchant. Hydrofluoric acid (HF) reacts with the silicon dioxide on the surface of glass ceramics and dissolves it.

$$4HF + SiO_2 = SiF_4 \uparrow + 2H_2O$$

Due to the different acid resistance of the crystalline phase and the glass phase in glass ceramics, the glass phase is more easily corroded by acid. Therefore, after glass ceramics are etched by hydrofluoric acid, the surface forms a honeycomb-like structure which is uneven, facilitating mechanical fixation. After etching, it should be rinsed with plenty of water, preferably with ultrasonic cleaning, to completely remove the hydrofluoric acid and the reaction products adhering to the ceramic surface.

After hydrofluoric acid etching, the glass-ceramic surface is rich in Si-OH, which easily reacts with silane coupling agents (such as 3-methacryloxy propyl trimethoxyl silane (MPS)) to form -Si-O- chemical bonds. The methyl methacrylate ester bond at the other end of the silane coupling agent can polymerize with acrylic acid resin adhesives, ultimately forming a chemical bond between the adhesive and the glass-ceramic (Fig. 6).

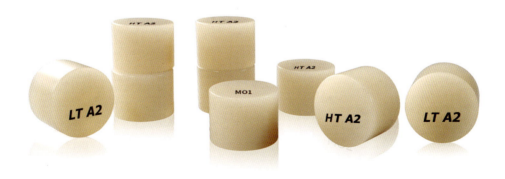

6

6 热压铸玻璃陶瓷
Hot isostatic pressing of glass ceramics

第3节　树脂基陶瓷

Section 3 Resin-based Ceramics

概述及分类

1. 概述

树脂基陶瓷是一种特殊类型的复合材料，由树脂基体与陶瓷颗粒、纤维或其他形态的陶瓷材料结合而成。树脂基陶瓷严格意义上不属于陶瓷，不能烧结加工，但由于树脂基陶瓷的力学性能和美学性能与陶瓷材料接近，适应证也类似，也可视为全瓷材料的一类。这种复合材料将树脂的可塑性和陶瓷的强度、硬度、耐磨性等特性结合在一起，具有独特的性能优势（图7）。

2. 分类

可切削树脂基陶瓷按制备工艺一般可分为混合法制备的可切削复合树脂陶瓷和渗透法制备的可切削树脂渗透陶瓷，混合法是将单体与填料混合，经过干燥、成型、固化形成最终的可切削树脂基陶瓷；渗透法需要先预制陶瓷骨架，然后渗透树脂单体，最后进行固化。

Overview and classification

1. Overview

Resin-based ceramics are a special type of composite material, composed of a resin matrix combined with ceramic particles, fibers, or other forms of ceramic materials. Strictly speaking, resin-based ceramics do not belong to ceramics, cannot undergo sintering processes, but due to their mechanical and aesthetic properties being similar to ceramic materials, and their indications also being similar, they can also be considered a type of all-ceramic material. This composite material combines the plasticity of resin with the strength, hardness, and abrasion resistance of ceramics, bringing unique performance advantages (Fig. 7).

2. Classification

The resin-based ceramic that can be cut can be divided into machinable composite resin ceramics prepared by mixing method and machinable resin infiltration ceramics prepared by infiltration method. The mixing method involves mixing monomers with fillers, drying, shaping, and curing to form the final machinable resin-based ceramic; the infiltration method requires a prefabricated ceramic framework first, then infiltrating with resin monomers, and finally curing.

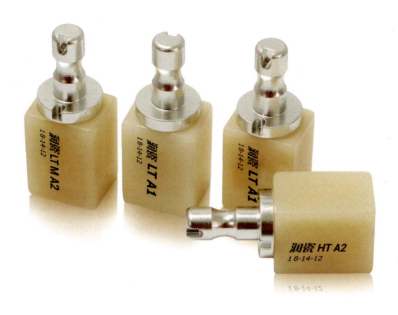

7

7 树脂基陶瓷
Resin-based ceramics

树脂基陶瓷化学成分（表6）

表6 树脂基陶瓷化学成分

树脂聚合物	13%～43%
无机填料	55%～85%
添加剂	<1%
着色剂	<1%

　　树脂基陶瓷的填料一般使用微纳米颗粒（0.1～10μm），固含量可达80%，通常采用大小颗粒级配的复合填料方式，这种方式填料可提高力学性能，小颗粒在打磨、磨损过程中会磨损或脱落，形成的凹陷尺度小于光线波长，使表面保持光滑和光泽，凸显出优异的抛光性能和保持表面光滑性能。

Chemical composition of resin-based ceramics (Table 6)

Table 6 Chemical Composition of Resin-based Ceramics

Resin polymer	13%-43%
Inorganic filler	55%-85%
Additive	<1%
Colorant	<1%

　　The fillers of resin-based ceramics generally use micro-nano particles (0.1-10 μm), with a solid content of up to 80%. Usually, a composite filler method with a size-graded distribution of particles is adopted. This method of filling can enhance the mechanical properties. Small particles will wear or detach during grinding and abrasion processes, forming depressions with scales smaller than the wavelength of light, which helps maintain a smooth and glossy surface, highlighting excellent polishing performance and maintaining surface smoothness.

理化性能（表7）

表7 树脂基陶瓷理化性能

弯曲强度	≥180MPa
抗压强度	≥350MPa
弹性模量	10~25GPa
吸水值	≤25g/mm^2
溶解值	≤7.5μg/mm^3

优缺点

1. 优点

效率：修复体制备过程不需要烧结，适合椅旁数字化修复。

美观性：树脂基陶瓷可以与自然牙齿颜色相匹配，提供良好的美观效果，使修复后的牙齿看起来更加自然。

弹性模量：弹性模量接近天然牙本质，适合种植上部结构，能起到吸收应力保护种植体的作用。

粘接性：树脂基陶瓷能够与牙体组织形成良好的粘接，降低了修复体脱落的风险。

2. 缺点

耐磨性较差：相对于其他全瓷材料，树脂基陶瓷的耐磨性较差，容易出现磨损和破损。

寿命较短：虽然树脂基陶瓷在修复后的牙齿上具有良好的美观效果，但其寿命相对较短，通常需要更频繁地更换。

Physical and chemical properties (Table 7)

Table 7 Properties of Resin-based Ceramics

Bending strength	≥180MPa
Compressive strength	≥350MPa
Elasticity modulus	10-25GPa
Water absorption	≤25 g/mm^2
Solubility	≤7.5μ g/mm^3

Advantages and disadvantages

1. Advantages

Efficiency: The repair system preparation process does not require sintering, which is suitable for chairside digital repair.

Appearance: Resin-based ceramics can match the color of natural teeth, providing good aesthetic results and making restored teeth look more natural.

Elastic modulus: The elastic modulus is close to the natural tooth structure, is suitable for implanting upper structures, and can absorb stress to protect the implant.

Adhesion: Resin-based ceramics can form good adhesion with dental tissues, reducing the risk of restoration detachment.

2. Disadvantages

Poor wear resistance: Compared to other all-ceramic materials, resin-based ceramics have poor wear resistance, making them prone to wear and damage.

Short lifespan: Although resin-based ceramics provide excellent aesthetic results on restored teeth, their lifespan is relatively short, often requiring more frequent replacement.

临床应用

嵌体、高嵌体、贴面、单冠（适合种植上部结构）。

应用指导

扫描模型获取、排版设计、加工、打磨抛光。

粘接

对于可切削树脂渗透陶瓷，氢氟酸酸蚀可以使表面陶瓷网络结构溶解，暴露树脂网络更有利于树脂水门汀的浸润铺展，增强微机械锁合力。与玻璃陶瓷相似，清洗后需涂布含硅烷偶联剂的底涂剂，硅烷偶联剂可与树脂渗透陶瓷中的二氧化硅形成化学性结合。

对于可切削复合树脂，多采用喷砂处理，喷砂压力常较小，一般小于0.2MPa以下。氢氟酸能部分溶解玻璃填料颗粒，形成微小凹坑，因此也可用氢氟酸蚀刻修复体粘接面。粗化处理完成后的修复体表面需要涂布树脂粘接剂，树脂粘接剂中的单体可以与树脂基质形成化学性结合。

Clinical application

Inlay, onlay, veneer, and single crown (suitable for implant superstructures).

Application guide

Scanning model acquisition, layout design, processing, polishing and finishing.

Adhesion

For machinable resin infiltrated ceramics, hydrofluoric acid etching can dissolve the surface ceramic network structure, exposing the resin network for better resin infiltration and spreading, enhancing the micro-mechanical interlocking force. Similar to glass ceramics, a primer containing silane coupling agent needs to be applied after cleaning, as the silane coupling agent can chemically bond with the silicon dioxide in the resin infiltrated ceramics.

Sandblasting is often used for machinable composite resins, with the pressure typically less than 0.2 MPa. Hydrofluoric acid can partially dissolve the glass filler particles, creating small pits, making it suitable for etching the bonding surface of restorations. After roughening treatment, the surface of the restoration needs to be coated with resin adhesive, and the monomers in the resin adhesive can chemically bond with the resin matrix.

第4节　聚甲基丙烯酸甲酯

Section 4 Polymethyl Methacrylate

概述

聚甲基丙烯酸甲酯，简称ＰＭＭＡ，俗称有机玻璃或亚克力。是由甲基丙烯酸甲酯（MMA）经自由基聚合而生成的一种热塑性树脂。ＰＭＭＡ为无定型聚合物，具有很多优良性能，如化学稳定性好，物理机械性能较均衡，表观光泽性、透明度及后加工性能良好，是一种综合性能优异的透明材料。PMMA被广泛应用于牙科领域，用于制作基牙、模型、义齿、种植导板等（图8）。

成分和性能

1. 成分

聚甲基丙烯酸甲酯（PMMA）是一种常见的合成树脂，其组成主要是由甲基丙烯酸甲酯单体（也称为甲基丙烯酸甲酯）组成。这种单体是通过化学反应将甲基丙烯酸与甲醇进行缩聚而成。其化学结构如下：

$$[-CH_2-C(CH_3)(COOCH_3)-]$$

Overview

Polymethyl methacrylate, abbreviated as PMMA and commonly known as acrylic or plexiglass, is a thermoplastic resin produced by the free radical polymerization of methyl methacrylate (MMA). PMMA is widely used in various applications due to its transparency, impact resistance, and UV stability. PMMA is an amorphous polymer with many excellent properties, such as good chemical stability, relatively balanced physical and mechanical properties, good surface gloss, transparency, and post-processing properties, making it an excellent transparent material. PMMA is widely used in the field of dentistry for making denture bases, models, dentures, and implant guides (Fig. 8).

Composition and properties

1. Composition

Polymethyl methacrylate (PMMA) is a common synthetic resin, primarily composed of methyl methacrylate monomer. This monomer is synthesized by the condensation reaction of methyl methacrylate acid with methanol. Its chemical structure is as follows:

$$[-CH_2-C(CH_3)(COOCH_3)-]$$

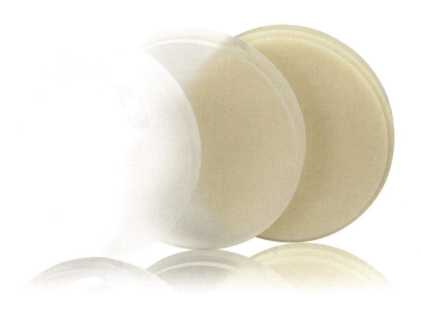

8

8 聚甲基丙烯酸甲酯
Polymethyl methacrylate

其中，[CH₂]表示甲基基团，[C(CH₃)]表示丙烯基团，[COOCH₃]表示甲酯基团。

[CH$_2$] represents the methyl group, [C(CH$_3$)] represents the propyl group, and [COOCH$_3$] represents the methyl ester group.

2. 理化性能（表8）

2. Physical and chemical properties (Table 8)

表8 PMMA性能

性能	参数
弯曲强度	≥50MPa
吸水值	≤40μg/mm^3
溶解值	≤7.5μg/mm^3

Table 8 PMMA Properties

Properties	Parameters
Bending strength	≥50MPa
Water absorption	≤40μg/mm^3
Solubility	≤7.5μg/mm^3

优缺点

1. 优点

透明度高：PMMA具有非常高的透明度，比玻璃还要透明，达到92%的透光率，使其成为制造透明产品的理想选择。

低密度：PMMA的密度较低，为1.19～1.20g/cm³，轻巧而不沉重，使其在制造轻量化产品时具有优势。

加工性能好：PMMA易于加工和成型，可以通过注塑、挤出、压延等方法制造出各种形状和尺寸的产品。

耐化学腐蚀性好：PMMA对大多数常见的化学品具有较好的耐腐蚀性，不易受到酸碱等化学物质的侵蚀。

2. 缺点

机械性能较差：PMMA的机械强度相对较低，抗冲击性和抗划伤性较差，容易发生断裂或划痕。

热稳定性较差：PMMA的热稳定性较差，容易在高温条件下软化、变形或分解，因此在高温环境中的应用受到限制。

易受溶剂影响：PMMA对某些有机溶剂敏感，容易受到溶剂的溶解和膨胀，导致尺寸变化或损坏。

临床应用

临时冠桥、种植导板、咬合夹板等。

Advantages and disadvantages

1. Advantages

High transparency: PMMA has a very high level of transparency, even higher than glass, with a light transmittance of up to 92%, making it an ideal choice for manufacturing transparent products.

Low density: PMMA has a density of approximately 1.19-1.20 g/cm³, making it lightweight and advantageous for manufacturing lightweight products.

Good processing performance: PMMA is easy to process and shape, and can be manufactured into products of various shapes and sizes through methods such as injection molding, extrusion, and rolling.

Good chemical corrosion resistance - PMMA has good resistance to most common chemicals and is not easily corroded by acids, alkalis, and other chemical substances.

2. Disadvantages

Poor mechanical performance: PMMA has relatively low mechanical strength, poor impact resistance, and scratch resistance, and is prone to fracture or scratching.

Poor thermal stability: PMMA exhibits poor thermal stability, making it prone to softening, deformation, or decomposition under high temperature conditions, thereby limiting its application in high temperature environments.

Easily affected by solvents, PMMA is sensitive to certain organic solvents. It can be easily dissolved and expanded by solvents, which can lead to dimensional changes or damage.

Clinical applications

Temporary crown bridge, planting guide plate, occlusal splint, etc.

应用指导

1. 加工

将临时冠桥树脂块按口腔修复技术常规操作的方法放到CAD/CAM机器中，按系统说明书指示的操作顺序用研磨钻加工临时冠桥树脂块。机械加工完成后，将树脂块从CAD/CAM机器中移出，用金刚石磨具将切削完成的冠、桥结构从临时冠桥树脂块中切削下来。

2. 抛光

修复体可以用合适的硅树脂抛光剂和小山羊毛刷进行预抛光。为了避免菌斑的积累和其他相关的对阴影的负面影响，仔细地抛光是绝对必要的。

3. 清洁

将完成的修复体放入超声波装置中约1分钟。碱性清洗液的含量不超过10%，温度不超过40℃，避免用蒸汽和压应力清洗。

4. 粘接

粘接前首先需要对PMMA表面进行适当的处理，以提高其表面活性和粗糙度，增强粘接剂与PMMA的结合力。通常采用机械打磨或溶剂溶胀法进行处理，聚甲基丙烯酸甲酯树脂可用牙托水（甲基丙烯酸甲酯，MMA）或氯仿进行溶胀。粗化后应选择与PMMA表面相容性良好的粘接剂，如甲基丙烯酸酯类粘接剂。

Application guide

1. Processing

The temporary crown and bridge resin blocks are placed in the CAD/CAM machine according to conventional procedures of dental restoration techniques. The resin blocks are processed with a milling bur according to the instructions in the manual. Once the mechanical processing is completed, the resin blocks are removed from the CAD/CAM machine, and the finished crown and bridge structures are cut out from the temporary crown and bridge resin blocks using diamond burs.

2. Polishing

Pre-polishing of the repaired body can be done with suitable silicone polishing agents and a small goat hairbrush. Careful polishing is necessary to avoid the accumulation of plaque and other related negative effects on the shade.

3. Cleaning

Place the completed repair in the ultrasonic unit for about 1 minute. The alkaline cleaning solution should not exceed 10%, the temperature should not exceed 40°C, and avoid using steam and pressure for cleaning.

4. Adhesion

Before adhesion, the PMMA surface needs to be properly treated to enhance its surface activity and roughness, thereby strengthening the bond between the adhesive and PMMA. Typically, mechanical grinding or solvent swelling methods are used for treatment, and polymethyl methacrylate resin can be swelled with dental impressions (methyl methacrylate, MMA) or chloroform. After roughening, an adhesive with good compatibility with the PMMA surface, such as methacrylate adhesive, should be selected.

临床病例实践

CLINICAL PRACTICE

病例1 数字化全程导板引导下双侧尖牙种植术中口扫即刻过渡修复一例

Case 1 Digital Template of Full–guided Implant Insertion with Immediate Interim Restorations for Bilateral Canines: A Case Report

本病例资料由张振生医生、刘海林技师提供，余涛医生整理
Provided from Dr. Zhensheng Zhang and Dt. Hailin Liu, and arranged by Dr. Tao Yu

初诊情况

基本信息：25岁男性。

主诉：双侧上颌尖牙先天缺失。

现病史：患者双侧上颌尖牙先天缺失，影响美观，现已通过正畸治疗调整缺牙间隙，要求种植修复，并尽快恢复美观。否认烟酒嗜好。

既往史：体健。

检查：13、23缺失，黏膜无明显红肿，近远中间隙及咬合间隙基本正常。13牙槽嵴唇侧轻度吸收，唇侧高度、丰满度少量下降；23牙槽嵴高度、丰满度均无明显下降。14、12、22、24无明显缺损，叩痛（－），不松动，牙龈无红肿（图2~图6）。

中位笑线，微笑时前牙区牙龈暴露量较少（图1）。

影像学检查：CBCT显示13、23牙槽骨高度充足，宽度为5~6mm，牙槽嵴向唇侧倾斜角度较大。

Pretreatment

Basic information: 25-year-old male.

Chief complaint: Bilateral congenital absence of maxillary canines.

History of present illness: The patient had bilateral congenital absence of maxillary canines, which affected the appearance. The gaps of the missing teeth were adjusted by orthodontic treatment. He asked for implant restoration to improve the appearance as soon as possible. Smoking and alcohol addiction were denied.

Past history: In good health.

Examination: Tooth 13 and 23 were missing. The mucosa had no obvious redness and swelling. Mesiodistal space and occlusal space were adequate. The labial side of the alveolar ridge of tooth 13 was slightly absorbed, resulting in a slight decreasing of the height and fullness. The height and fullness of the alveolar ridge of tooth 23 showed no obvious decreasing. For tooth 14, 12, 22, 24, there was no obvious defect, no percussion pain, no mobility, and no redness or swelling of the gingiva (Figs. 2 to 6).

He had a median smile line with a little gingival exposing in the anterior region when smiling (Fig. 1).

Radiographic examination: CBCT showed that the alveolar bone of bilateral edentulous area was sufficient in height and about 5 to 6mm in width, with a large angle of inclination of the alveolar ridge to the labial side.

诊断

上颌牙列缺损。

治疗计划

方案一：13种植+植骨，5个月后二期手术，必要时结缔组织移植，1~3个月后过渡修复，1.5个月后永久修复；23种植+即刻修复，与13同时永久修复。

方案二：13、23种植+即刻修复，3个月后永久修复。

考虑到患者中位笑线，牙龈暴露量少，且尽量减少创伤、尽快恢复美观意愿强烈，与患者协商后决定适当妥协13的粉色美学效果，按照方案二进行治疗，并且采用数字化全程导板引导下不翻瓣微创种植。

术前准备

制取口内数字印模，并与术前CBCT一并导入种植导板设计软件，在13、23分别设计植入一颗Bredent SKY3.5mm×14mm种植体（图7~图11），完成全程种植导板设计。3D打印上颌模型（图12），打印种植导板并粘接金属导环（图13）。模型上试戴导板，贴合、稳定、固位力良好（图14），试引导型种植体携带器与导环密合（图15），准备种植导板手术工具盒（图16）。

Diagnosis

Maxillary dentition defect.

Treatment plan

Plan 1: For tooth 13, implant and bone grafting, the second stage operation with possible soft tissue augmentation 5 months later, interim restoration 1-3 months later, definitive restoration 1.5 months later; for tooth 23, implant with immediate restoration, definitive restoration at the same time with tooth 13.

Plan 2: For both tooth 13 and 23, implant with immediate restoration, and definitive restoration 3 months later.

Considering the patient's median smile line, less gingival exposure, and strong desire to reduce trauma as much as possible to restore the appearance as soon as possible, we decided to compromise the pink aesthetic effect of 13 after consultation with the patient, and the treatment was carried out according to plan 2, and the digital full-guided template was used to guide the flapless minimally invasive implant placement.

Preoperative preparation

The intraoral digital impressions were taken and imported into the implant guide design software together with preoperative CBCT. Two Bredent SKY 3.5×14mm implants was designed and implanted on 13 and 23 (Figs. 7 to 11) to complete the whole implant guide design. The maxillary model was printed by 3D printing (Fig. 12), and the implant guide template was printed and bonded with the metal guide ring (Fig. 13). The template was fitted on the model with good fit, stability, and retention (Fig. 14). The guided implant driver was fitted well with the guide ring (Fig. 15), and the surgical toolbox of the guided implant placement was prepared (Fig. 16).

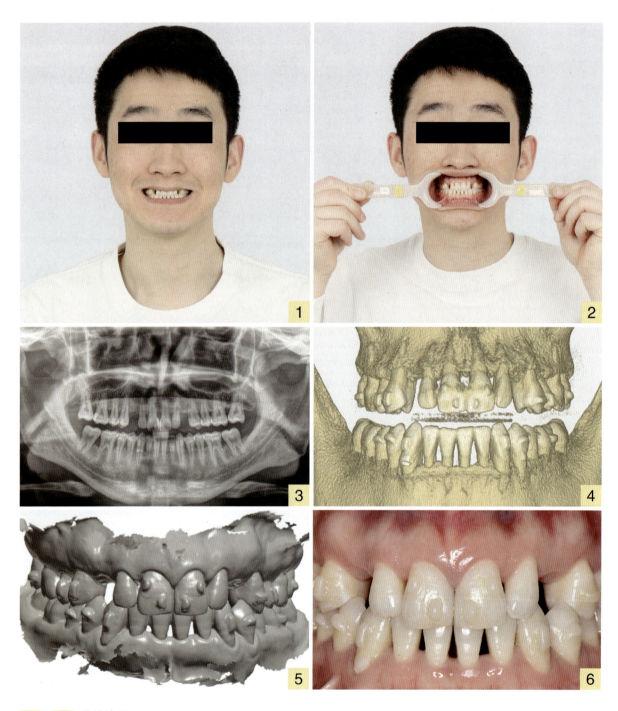

1 ~ 6 术前检查
Pretreatment examination

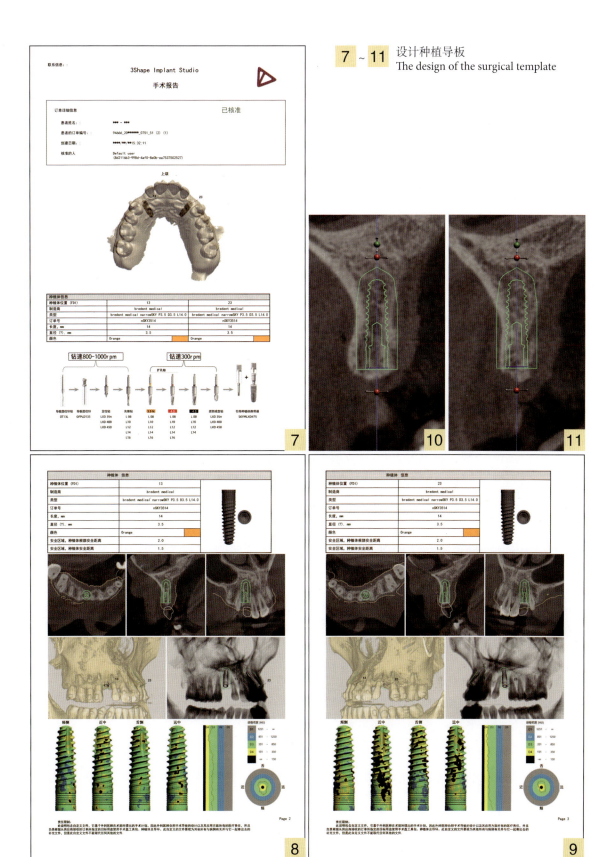

7 ~ 11 设计种植导板
The design of the surgical template

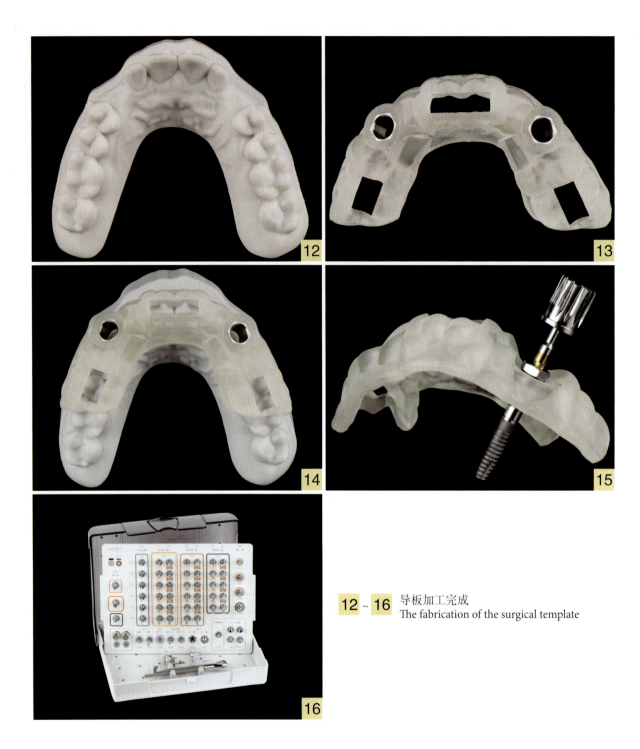

12 ~ 16 导板加工完成
The fabrication of the surgical template

治疗过程

术前于患者口内试戴导板，就位之后导板稳定、固位力良好，从观察窗确认导板贴合（图17和图18）。

常规消毒铺巾后，13、23局麻。再次确认导板完全就位（图25），导板引导下自8mm先锋钻开始，预备至14mm先锋钻完全进入导板，止动环与导环接触（图26和图27）。探查确认洞壁完整（图28）。之后依次进行扩孔钻、颈部成型钻预备（图29～图31）。取出种植体，并安装引导型种植体携带器，上紧至10Ncm（图32和图33），导板引导下植入种植体，直至携带器止动环与导环完全接触，止动环六边形结构与导环六边形完全重叠，植入扭矩约45Ncm（图34～图37）。种植体植入后牙槽嵴顶仅有一个较小的圆形切口（图38），且由于牙槽嵴顶并非完全平整，种植体周围牙槽骨存在影响修复基台就位的可能，因此再使用骨成型钻修整种植体周围牙槽骨（图39）。以相同方式完成两颗种植体的植入（图19），并修整对应种植体周围牙槽骨（图20），安装愈合基台（图21）。拍摄CBCT，显示种植体位置良好（图22～图24）。

基于"one-abutment-one-time"的理念，修复体将采取个性化基台+全冠的形式，永久修复时仅更换全冠，而不更换也不取下个性化基台。13、23取下愈合基台，安装扫描杆并确认就位（图40），制取口内数字印模，设计即刻过渡修复体。数字化设计个性化基台（图41），在其之上设计全冠，切削Bio-HPP个性

Treatment process

The template was fitted intraorally before operation and was stable with good retention after placement. The fit of the template was confirmed from the observation windows (Figs. 17 and 18).

After routine disinfection, local anesthesia was applied for tooth 13 and 23. The template was reconfirmed fully in place (Fig. 25). Under the guidance of the template, pioneer drilling started from the 8mm pioneer bur to the 14mm one. Each bur completely entered the template, and the stopper contacted the guide ring (Figs. 26 and 27). A probe was used to confirm that the hole wall was intact (Fig. 28). After that, reaming drill and neck shaping drill preparation were performed in turn (Figs. 29 to 31). The guided implant driver was installed on the implant and tight to 10Ncm (Figs. 32 and 33). Under the guidance of the template, the implant was placed until the stopper of the driver was completely in contact with the guide ring, the hexagonal structure of the stopper was completely overlapped with the hexagonal structure of the guide ring, and the insertion torque was about 45Ncm (Figs. 34 to 37). After implant placement, there was only a small circular incision at the alveolar crest (Fig. 38). Because the alveolar crest was not completely flat, the alveolar bone around the implant might affect the placement of the abutment, so the bone molding drill was used to reduce the alveolar bone around the implant (Fig. 39). The two implants were implanted in the same way (Fig. 19), the corresponding alveolar bone around the implants was adjusted (Fig. 20), and the healing abutment was installed (Fig. 21). CBCT was taken and showed that the implants were in good position (Figs. 22 to 24).

Based on the "one-abutment-one-time" concept, the restorations would take the form of personalized abutments with full crowns, and only the full crowns would be replaced for the definitive restorations, without replacing or removing the personalized abutment. The healing abutments were removed, and the scanning posts were installed and confirmed to be in place (Fig. 40). Then the digital intraoral impression was taken to design the immediate interim restoration. The personalized abutments were digitally designed (Fig.

化基台与复合树脂全冠（图42），逐级打磨抛光，完成即刻过渡修复体制作（图43）。口内试戴个性化基台，牙龈形态基本协调，全冠修复体空间合适，上紧中央螺丝至25Ncm（图44），暂封螺丝孔。全冠就位后与对颌牙、邻牙均没有接触，使用临时粘接剂将其粘接于个性化基台之上，完成即刻过渡修复（图45），拍摄X线片确认修复体完全就位（图48）。通过种植体植入+即刻过渡修复体，快速恢复了患者前牙美观（图46和图47）。术后验证显示，13、23种植体植入角度误差分别为1.37°、1.36°，根尖误差分别为0.42mm、0.46mm（图49和图50）。

即刻修复2周后复查，手术伤口愈合良好，黏膜无明显红肿，过渡修复体、种植体无松动（图51～图54）。即刻修复3个月后，软组织状态稳定，无明显红肿（图55）。取下临时粘接的复合树脂全冠，个性化基台加力至25Ncm，聚四氟乙烯膜+流动树脂封闭螺丝孔（图56和图57），制取基台水平硅橡胶印模（图58和图59），比色A1～A2（图60）。灌制石膏工作模型（图61），分离代型，制作全冠蜡型（图62），使用热压铸锂瓷制作铸瓷全冠，逐级打磨抛光（图63），在模型上试戴合适后（图64），染色上釉完成全冠制作（图65）。

41), and the full crowns were designed on top of them. The Bio-HPP personalized abutments and the composite resin full crowns were milled (Fig. 42) and polished step by step to complete the immediate interim restorations (Fig. 43). After the personalized abutments were tried in the mouth, the shapes of the gingiva were basically coordinated, and the space of the full crowns were suitable. The central screws were tightened to 25Ncm (Fig. 44), and the screw holes were sealed temporarily. After the full crowns were placed in place, there were no contact of them with the opposite teeth or adjacent teeth. The temporary adhesive was used to bond the full crowns to the personalized abutments to complete the immediate interim restorations (Fig. 45). X-ray films were taken to confirm that the restorations were completely in place (Fig. 48). The appearance of the patient's anterior teeth was quickly restored through implants placement and immediate interim restorations (Figs. 46 and 47). Postoperative verification showed that the angle errors of implants 13 and 23 were 1.37° and 1.36°, respectively, and the apical errors were 0.42mm and 0.46mm, respectively (Figs. 49 and 50).

Two weeks after the immediate restoration, the surgical wound healed well, the mucosa did not show obvious redness and swelling, and there was no loosening of the interim restorations and implants (Figs. 51 to 54). Three months after the immediate restoration, the soft tissue condition was stable without obvious redness and swelling (Fig. 55). The temporarily bonded composite resin crowns were removed, and the personalized abutments were tightened to 25Ncm. The screw holes were closed with PTFE membrane and flowable resin (Figs. 56 and 57). The abutment level silicone impression was made (Figs. 58 and 59), and the colors of the teeth were between A1 and A2 (Fig. 60). The plaster working model (Fig. 61) was filled, the generation model was separated, and the wax model of the full crowns were made (Fig. 62). The hot-pressed lithium disilicate ceramic was used to make the full crowns, which were polished step by step (Fig. 63). Fitting on the model (Fig. 64), the full crowns were finally completed after dyeing and glazing (Fig. 65).

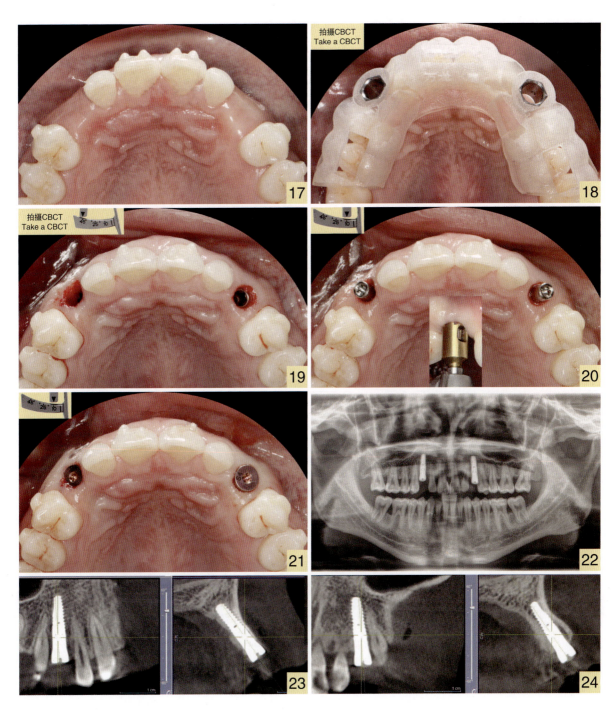

17 ~ 24　术中概览
Overview of the surgery

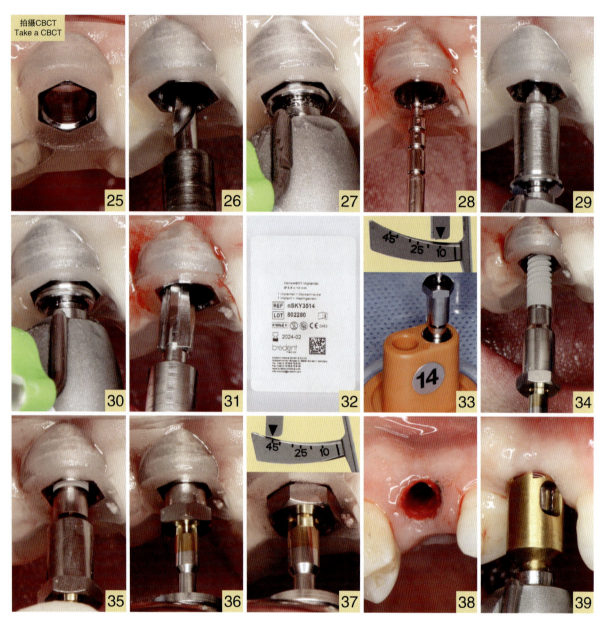

25 ~ 39 术中细节
Details of the surgery

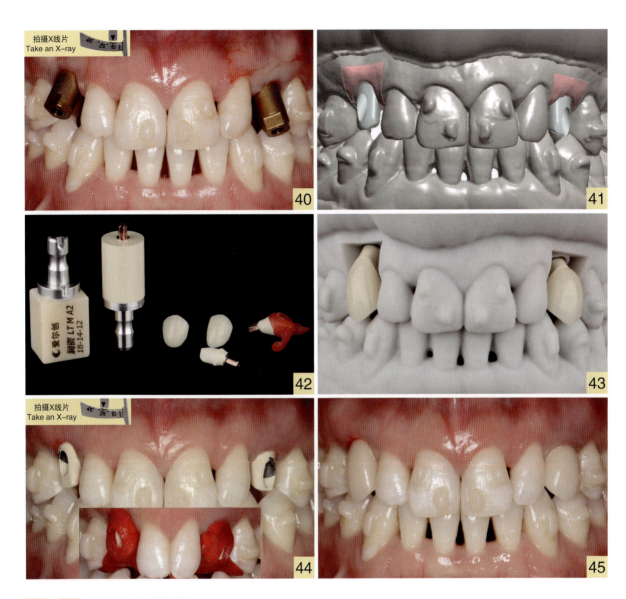

40 ~ 45 制作安装临时修复体
The procedure of the interim restorations

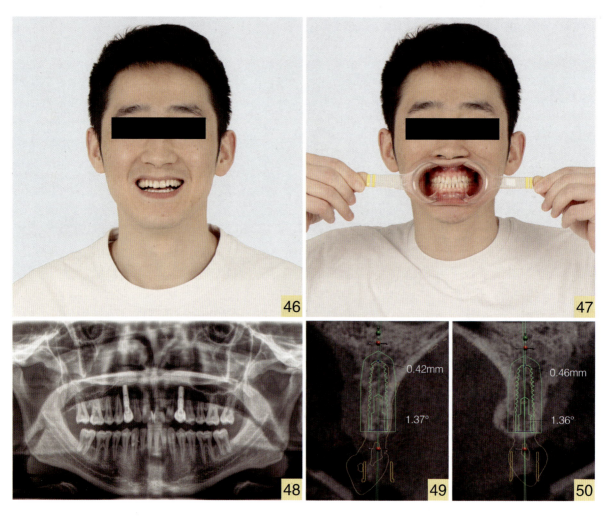

46 ~ 50　安装临时修复体
The results of the interim restorations

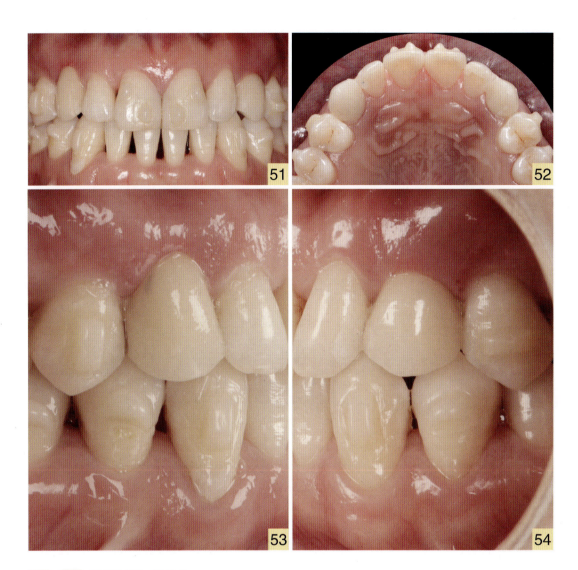

51 ~ 54 临时修复体2周复查
Two weeks after the delivery of the interim restorations

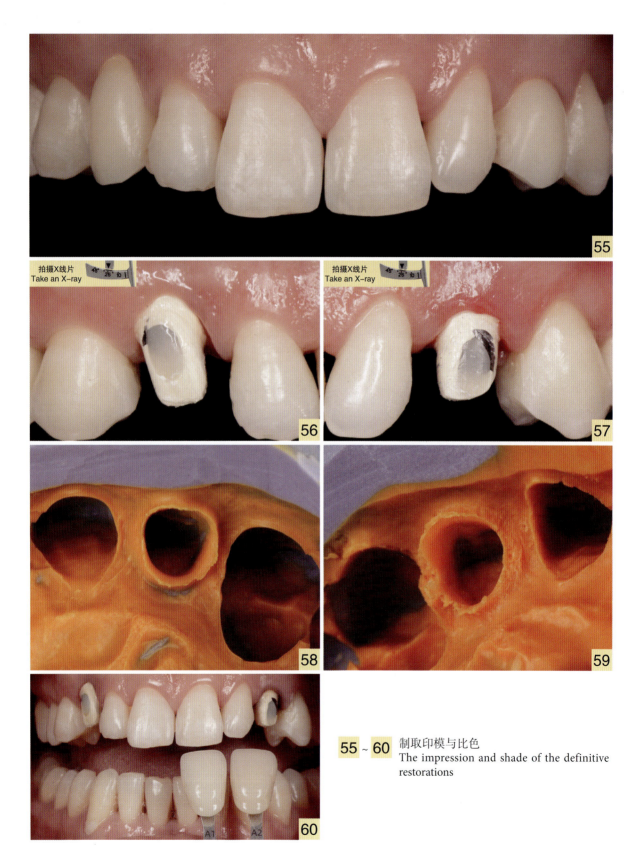

55 ~ 60 制取印模与比色
The impression and shade of the definitive restorations

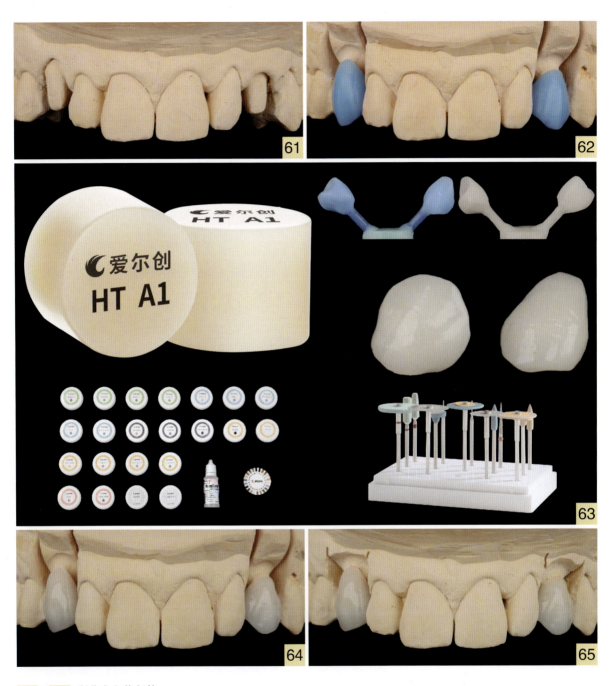

61 ~ 65 制作永久修复体
The procedure of the definitive restorations

取下复合树脂全冠后，试戴铸瓷全冠，调
殆，抛光，使用树脂水门汀粘接，并彻底清除
多余粘接剂（图66～图71）。戴牙后拍摄X线

After the composite resin full crowns were removed, the ceramic full crowns were fitted, adjusted, polished, bonded with resin cement, and the excessive cement was thoroughly removed (Figs. 66 to 71). The X-ray

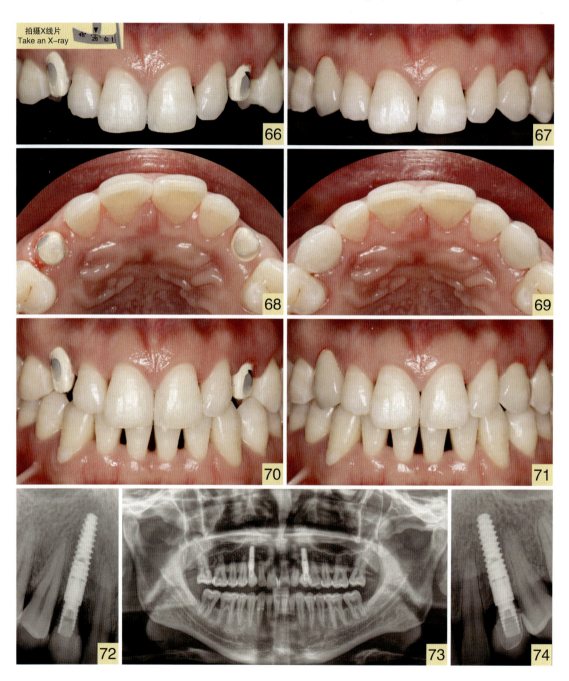

66 ~ 74 安装永久修复体
The delivery of the definitive restorations

片显示全冠完全就位，边缘密合，未见残余粘接剂（图72~图74）。13、23两颗修复体形态、颜色、质地自然，与患者天然牙协调，较明显地改善了患者的前牙美观效果。3个月后复查，修复体、种植体稳定，周围软组织无红肿（图75~图79）。

films taken after wearing the teeth showed that the full crowns were completely in place, the edges were fit, and no excessive cement was observed (Figs. 72 to 74). The two restorations of 13 and 23 had natural shape, color, and texture, which were in harmony with the patient's natural teeth, and significantly improved the patient's anterior teeth aesthetic effect. Three months later, the restorations and implants were stable, and there was no redness and swelling in the surrounding soft tissue (Figs. 75 to 79).

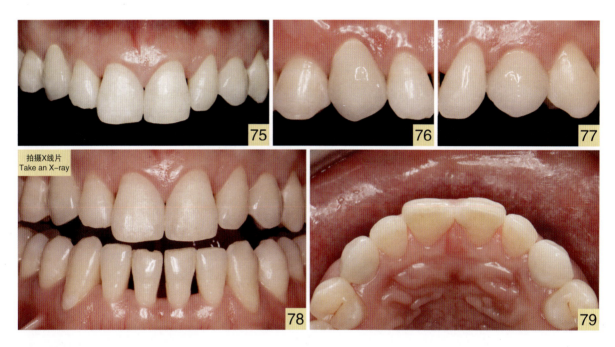

75 ~ 79 永久修复3个月后复查
Three months after the delivery of the definitive restorations

讨论

正确的种植体植入的位置、轴向是美学区种植治疗获得成功的重要前提之一。本病例缺牙区牙槽骨宽度仅5~6mm，且牙槽骨倾斜明显，对种植体植入的准确度要求较高。使用全程种植导板，可以有效提高种植体植入的准确度。既往研究表明，种植导板手术的植入角度误差为2°~5°，根尖误差为1~1.5mm。本病例两个种植位点的植入角度误差分别为1.37°、1.36°，根尖误差分别为0.42mm、0.46mm，达到了较高的准确度。

根据"one-abutment-one-time"的理念，种植术后即刻安装修复基台，并不再取下基台，不破坏软组织–基台连接界面，有利于保持软组织稳定。Bio-HPP是以PEEK为主的复合材料，具有良好的生物相容性，且加工方便，能快速完成即刻修复。本病例采用的Bio-HPP基台是通过热压铸的方式，将Bio-HPP压铸于钛基底之上，两种材料结合界面的强度较传统粘接界面有明显提高，可用于永久修复，且已有研究报道获得了良好的临床效果。

本病例通过数字化全程种植导板微创而准确地在前牙区植入两颗种植体，采用个性化Bio-HPP基台+复合树脂全冠快速完成即刻过渡修复，并最终将全冠更换为铸瓷全冠，获得较为协调、自然的美学效果。

Discussion

Correct placement and axial orientation of implants is one of the most important prerequisites for successful implant treatment in the esthetic zone. In this case, the width of the alveolar bone in the edentulous area was only 5-6 mm, and the alveolar bone was obviously inclined, which required high accuracy of implant placement. The use of full-guided template can effectively improve the accuracy of implant placement. According to previous studies, the angle error of implant guide surgery was about 2-5 °, and the apical error was about 1-1.5 mm. In this case, the Angle errors of the two implant sites were 1.37° and 1.36°, and the apical errors were 0.42mm and 0.46mm, respectively, which reached a high accuracy.

According to the concept of "one-abutment-one-time", the abutment can be installed immediately after implantation without removing the abutment and destroying the soft tissue-abutment connection interface, which is conducive to maintaining the stability of soft tissue. Bio-HPP is a composite material based on PEEK, which has good biocompatibility and easy processing, and can quickly complete the immediate restoration. The Bio-HPP abutment used in this case was cast on titanium base. The strength of the bonding interface between the two materials is significantly higher than that of the traditional bonding interface, which can be used for definitive restoration. Previous studies have reported good clinical results.

In this case, the digital implant template was used to minimally invasion and accurately place two implants in the anterior region, and the personalized Bio-HPP abutments and composite resin full crowns were used to quickly complete the immediate interim restorations. Finally, the full crowns were replaced by ceramics, and a more coordinated and natural aesthetic effect was obtained.

病例2 数字化全程导板引导后牙种植并置入术前预成即刻过渡修复体一例

Case 2 Digital Full-guided Template for Posterior Dental Implantations with Preoperative Fabricated Immediate Interim Restorations: A Case Report

本病例资料由吴华庭医生、刘海林技师提供，余涛医生整理

Provided from Dr. Huating Wu and Dt. Hailin Liu, and arranged by Dr. Tao Yu

初诊情况

基本信息：34岁女性。

主诉：左上后牙缺失3个月，右下后牙缺失3年余。

现病史：左上及右下各有一颗后牙分别于3个月和3年余以前，因缺损严重而拔除，现双侧后牙咀嚼均受影响，要求种植修复。否认烟酒嗜好。

既往史：体健。

检查：25、46缺失，牙槽嵴中度吸收，黏膜无明显红肿，角化黏膜宽度正常，近远中间隙及咬合间隙基本正常。

影像学检查：CBCT显示25缺牙区牙槽骨宽为7~8mm、高为11~12mm，腭侧牙槽骨少量吸收，骨质密度偏低，约为Ⅲ类骨；46缺牙区牙槽骨宽为6~8mm、高约15mm；牙槽嵴顶颊侧吸收明显，骨质密度中等，约为Ⅱ类骨。

Pretreatment

Basic information: 34-year-old female.

Chief complaint: The left upper posterior tooth was missing for 3 months and the right lower posterior tooth was missing for more than 3 years.

History of present illness: One upper left posterior tooth and one lower right posterior tooth were extracted because of severe defect 3 months and 3 years ago, respectively. Now chewing of bilateral posterior teeth was affected, and implant restorations were required. She denied any smoking or drinking habits.

Past history: In good health.

Examination: Tooth 25 and 46 were missing with moderate absorption of alveolar ridge, no obvious redness and swelling of mucosa, normal width of keratinized mucosa, and basically normal mesiodistal space and occlusal space.

Radiographic examination: CBCT showed that the width and height of the alveolar bone of tooth 25 were 7-8 mm and 11-12 mm, respectively. The alveolar bone on the palatal side was slightly absorbed, and the bone density was low, about Class III bone. The width of the alveolar bone of tooth 46 was about 6-8 mm, the height was about 15mm, the alveolar crest was obviously absorbed on the buccal side, and the bone density was medium, about the type II bone.

诊断

上下颌牙列缺损。

治疗计划

25、46种植修复。

为了提高种植准确性和尽量减少创伤，计划采用数字化全程导板引导下不翻瓣微创种植。

术前准备

制取口内数字印模，并与术前CBCT一并导入种植导板设计软件（图1～图4），在25、46分别虚拟设计一颗牙冠，再以修复体为导向分别设计植入Bredent SKY4.0mm × 10mm、4.5mm × 12mm种植体各一颗（图5～图9），完成全程种植导板设计并输出虚拟设计的种植体位置，依照此位置设计即刻过渡修复体的个性化基台和外冠。3D种植导板并粘接金属导环（图10），在模型上试戴导板、贴合、稳定、固位力良好（图11和图12）。切削Bio-HPP个性化基台和复合树脂外冠，使用临时粘接剂将二者粘接。在技工室，于模型上模拟全程导板引导下植入种植体（图13和图14），种植体位置准确，并能够顺利戴入预成即刻过渡修复体，制作硅橡胶戴牙导板（图16～图18）。准备种植导板手术工具盒（图15）。

Diagnosis

Maxillary and mandibular dentition defect.

Treatment plan

Implant restorations for tooth 25 and 46.

In order to improve implant accuracy and minimize trauma, flap-free minimally invasive implant surgery guided by template was planned.

Preoperative preparation

The intraoral digital impression was taken and imported into the implant guide design software together with the preoperative CBCT (Figs. 1 to 4). Crowns were designed at 25 and 46, respectively, and then Bredent SKY 4.0×10mm and 4.5×12mm implants were designed based on the prosthetics-oriented design (Figs. 5 to 9). The whole process of implant guide template design was completed, and the implant positions of the virtual design were output. According to this position, the personalized abutments and external crowns were designed. The 3D guided templates and metal guide rings were bonded (Fig. 10). When the guided templates were fitted on the model, the fit, stability, and retention force were good (Figs. 11 and 12). The Bio-HPP customized abutments and composite resin crowns were milled and bonded with temporary adhesive. In the laboratory, implants were placed under the guidance of the full-range guide template on the model (Figs. 13 and 14). The position of the implants was accurate, and the prefabricated immediate interim prosthesis could be successfully placed (Figs. 16 to 18). The surgical toolbox for guided surgery was prepared (Fig. 15).

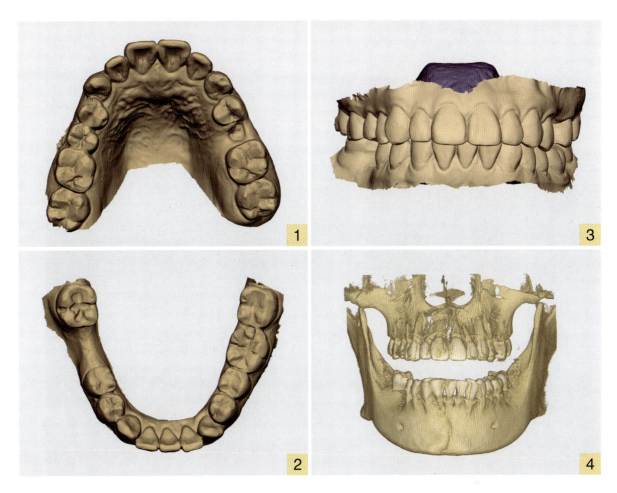

1 ~ 4 术前口内数字印模与CBCT
Preoperative intraoral impression and CBCT

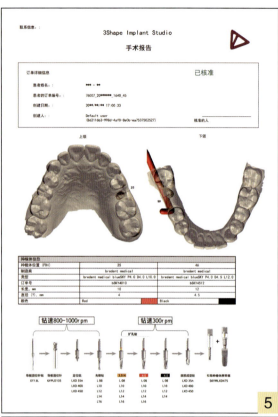

5~9 设计种植导板
The design of the surgical template

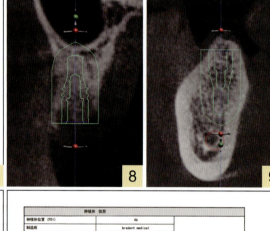

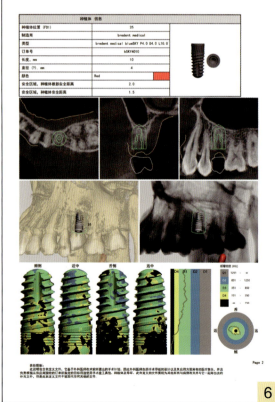

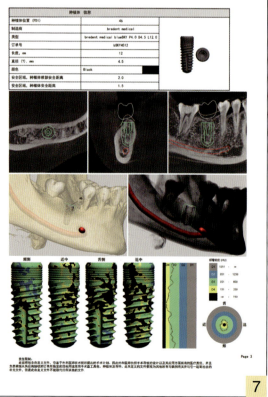

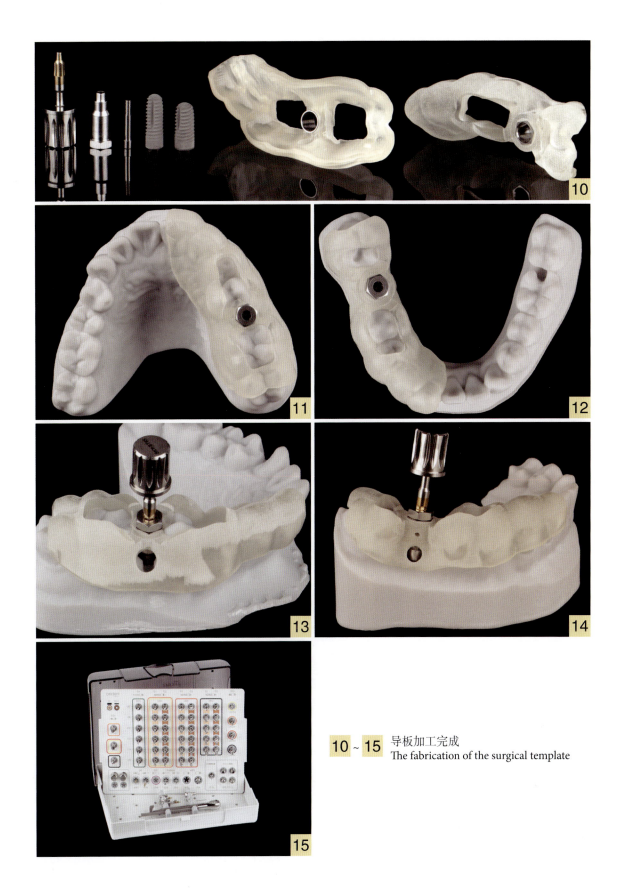

10 ~ 15 导板加工完成
The fabrication of the surgical template

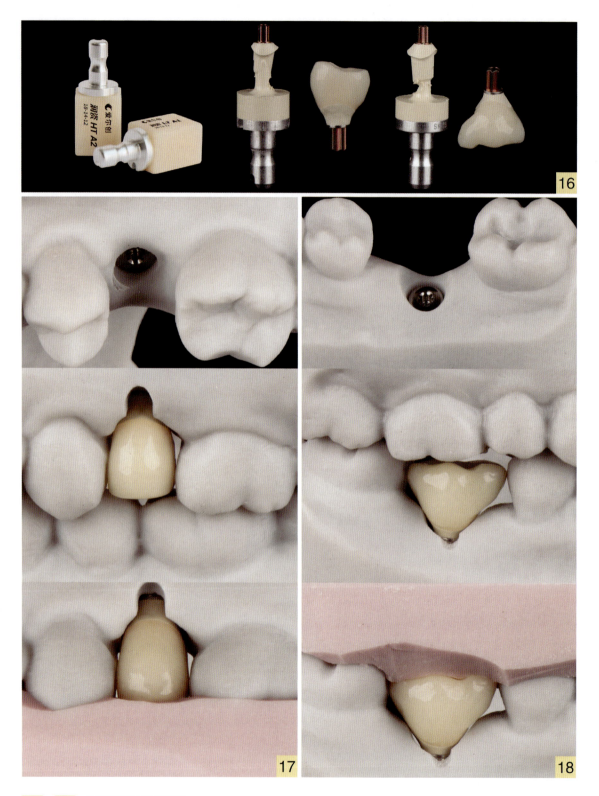

16 ~ **18** 术前制作过渡修复体

The preoperative fabrication of the interim restorations

治疗过程

　　术前于患者口内试戴导板，确认导板贴合、稳定、固位良好。常规消毒铺巾后，25局部浸润麻醉，再次确认导板完全就位（图19和图20），导板引导下牙龈环切打开手术入路（图21），定位钻定点避免后续钻针打滑或者跳钻（图22），8mm、10mm先锋钻先后下钻，确定备洞深度与方向（图23），降低钻速使用扩孔钻逐级扩孔至既定直径（图24和图25）。取出Bredent SKY4.0mm×10mm种植体，安装引导型种植体携带器，旋紧至10Ncm（图26和图27），导板引导下植入种植体，直至携带器止动环与导环完全接触，止动环六边形结构与导环六边形完全重叠，植入扭矩约45Ncm（图28和图29），取下引导型种植体携带器，再取下导板，见种植体位置良好（图30和图31）。硅橡胶戴牙导板辅助下安装即刻过渡修复体（图32和图33），为了尽可能减少愈合期种植体所受外力，修复体与对颌牙无咬合接触（图34），修复螺丝旋紧至25Ncm，树脂暂封螺丝孔（图35）。

　　46种植体植入与即刻过渡修复过程类似。待局部浸润麻醉后再次确认导板完全就位，导板引导下依次进行牙龈环切钻、定位钻、先锋钻、扩孔钻和颈部成型钻备洞，使用引导型种植体携带器植入Bredent SKY4.5mm×12mm种植体，安装即刻过渡修复体，避免咬合接触，旋紧至25Ncm，暂封螺丝孔（图38～图54）。

Treatment process

Before operation, it was confirmed that the guided templates were fit, stable, and well retained in the patient's mouth. After local anesthesia, the guide templates were put completely in place (Figs. 19 and 20). For tooth 25, the surgical approach began with the gingival ring incision guided by the guide template (Fig. 21). The point drill was used to avoid slip or skip of the following burs (Fig. 22). The pilot drill was used to determine the depth and direction of the hole preparation (Fig. 23). The reaming drills were used to gradually expand the hole to the planed diameter (Figs. 24 and 25). A Bredent SKY 4.0×10mm implant was connected to the guided implant carrier and tightened to 10Ncm (Figs. 26 and 27). The implant was placed under the guidance of the template until the stop ring of the carrier was completely in contact with the guide ring, and the hexagonal structure of the stop ring was completely overlapping with the hexagonal structure of the guide ring. The insertion torque was about 45Ncm (Figs. 28 and 29). The guided implant carrier was removed, and then the guide template was removed. The position of the implant was good (Figs. 30 and 31). The immediate transition prosthesis was installed with the assistance of a silicone rubber dental guide. (Figs. 32 and 33) In order to minimize the load on the implant during the healing period, there was no occlusal contact between the restoration and the opposite teeth (Fig. 34). The prosthetic screw was tightened to 25Ncm, and the screw holes was temporarily sealed by resin (Fig. 35).

The procedure of implant placement and immediate interim restoration was similar for tooth 46. A Bredent SKY 4.5×12mm implant was inserted under the guidance of the template and an immediate interim restoration was screwed (Figs. 38 to 54).

术后拍摄X线片显示25、46种植体位置良好，修复体完全就位（图36和图55）。术后验证种植准确度，25种植体植入角度误差1.07°，根尖区误差0.31mm；46种植体植入角度误差1.48°，根尖区误差0.38mm（图37和图56）。

3个月后，25、46过渡修复体及种植体无松动，黏膜无明显红肿，开始永久修复。先取下24过渡修复体，见软组织袖口内少量出血点，无明显炎症（图57），安装金属扫描杆，10Ncm旋紧（图58），制取25种植修复口内数字印模；以同样的方法取下46过渡修复体，安装金属扫描杆，制取46种植修复口内数字印模（图65和图66）。CAD软件中分别于25、46设计个性化修复基台（图59和图67），在基台上设计外冠（图60和图68）；分别切削Bio-HPP个性化基台、二硅酸锂全瓷外冠（图73和图74），外冠在基台上试戴合适后，进行抛光、烧结、染色上釉等一系列后处理，并用树脂水门汀粘接于基台之上（图75）。

临床试戴修复体，就位后近远中接触区松紧合适，旋紧修复螺丝至25Ncm，暂封螺丝孔（图61和图69），拍片确认修复体完全就位（图64和图72），使用流动树脂封闭螺丝孔，调𬌗，抛光（图62和图63、图70和图71）。完成25、46两个位置的种植修复，恢复缺牙区的咀嚼功能。

Postoperative X-ray films showed that 25, 46 implants were in good position and the restorations were completely in place (Figs. 36 and 55). The accuracy of implant placement was verified after operation. The Angle error of 25 implant was 1.07°, and the error in the apical area was 0.31mm. The Angle error of 46 implant was 1.48° and the error in the apical area was 0.38mm (Figs. 37 and 56).

Three months later, no loosening of the 25, 46 interim restorations and implants and no obvious redness and swelling of the mucosa were observed. Then the definitive restorations were started. A small amount of bleeding spots in the soft tissue cuff without obvious inflammation were observed (Fig. 57). A metal scanning post was installed and tightened at 10Ncm (Fig. 58). In the same way, the 46 interim restoration was removed, the metal scanning post was installed, and the intraoral digital impression was made (Figs. 65 and 66). The customized abutments (Figs. 59 and 67) and the external crowns (Figs. 60 and 68) were designed in CAD software. The Bio-HPP personalized abutments and lithium disilicates all-ceramic external crowns were milled respectively (Figs. 73 and 74). After fitting the outer crowns on the abutments, polishing, sintering, dyeing, glatening, and other post-treatments were performed, and the resin cement was bonded to the abutment (Fig. 75).

The proximal contacts of the crowns were proper. Then, the prosthetic screws were tightened to 25Ncm and the screw holes were sealed temporarily (Figs. 61 and 69). The X-ray films were taken to confirm that the restorations were completely in place (Figs. 64 and 72). The screw holes were closed with flowable resin. The occlusal adjustment and polishing were carried out later (Figs. 62, 63, 70, and 71). Implant restorations were completed at two positions 25 and 46 to restore the masticatory function of the missing tooth area.

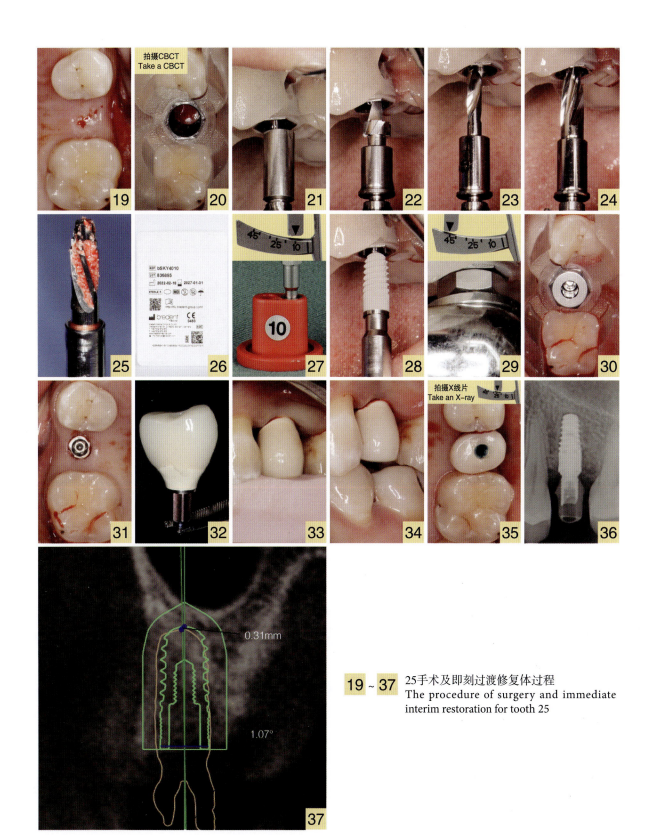

拍摄CBCT
Take a CBCT

拍摄X线片
Take an X-ray

19 ~ 37　25手术及即刻过渡修复体过程
The procedure of surgery and immediate interim restoration for tooth 25

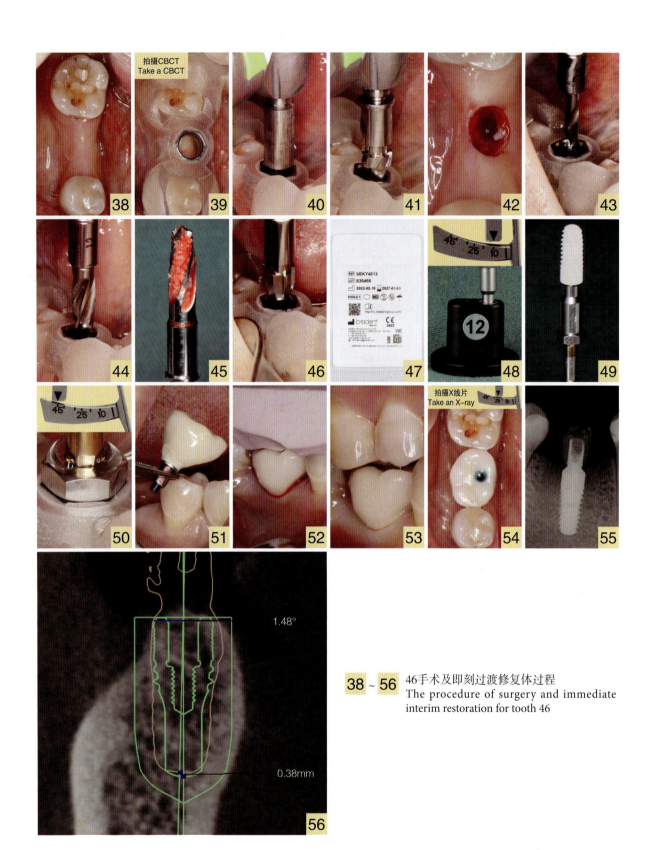

38 ~ 56 46手术及即刻过渡修复体过程
The procedure of surgery and immediate interim restoration for tooth 46

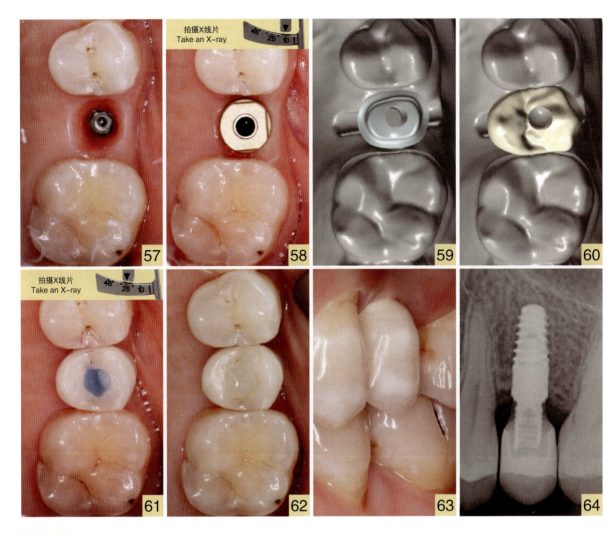

57 ~ 64 　25正式修复过程
The procedure of the definitive restoration for tooth 25

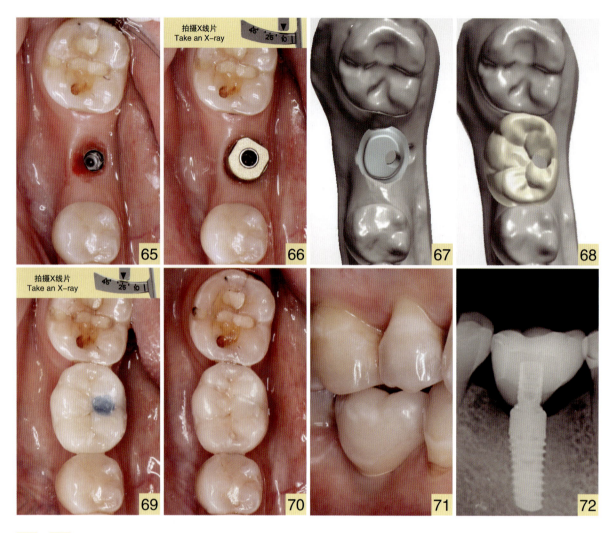

65 ~ **72** 46正式修复过程
The procedure of the definitive restoration for tooth 46

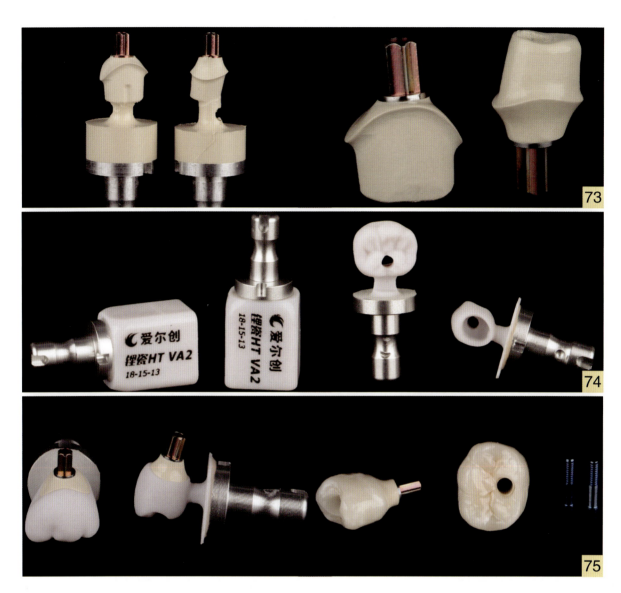

73 ~ 75 正式修复体的加工
The fabrication of the definitive restorations

讨论

后牙区正确的种植体植入的位置、角度，有利于种植体实行功能时的应力分散，降低不良应力带来的骨吸收及基台、螺丝或者种植体折断等风险。全程种植导板可较大提高种植体植入的准确度，即使在骨条件并不是特别充裕的情况下，同样可以实现不翻瓣微创种植。

本病例缺牙区牙槽嵴顶存在一定倾斜角度，钻针备洞时有打滑偏移的风险，先使用尖锐锋利的定位钻确定备洞中心点，可进一步提高备洞的准确度；在先锋钻和扩孔钻预备时，需要从最短的8mm钻开始，逐渐换钻加长至所需要的长度，保证钻针针尖接触牙槽骨时钻针引导结构已进入导环，起到引导作用。最终，25、46两个种植位点的植入角度误差分别为1.07°、1.48°，根尖误差分别为0.31mm、0.38mm，达到了较高的准确度。

为了保证术前预成即刻过渡修复体能够顺利就位，除了准确的种植体植入位置与角度，还需要准确控制种植体抗旋结构的旋转角度，也就是种植体沿其长轴方向自转的角度。这意味着必须使用全程导板，半程导板或先锋钻导板是无法控制种植体抗旋结构旋转角度的，目前的动态导航和种植机器人也无法保证正确的抗旋结构旋转角度。本病例先于技工室使用全程导板引导下，在模型上植入种植体的准确性，并顺利安装预成修复体，验证方法的有效性之后，再于临床成功开展对应手术与即刻过渡修复。

Discussion

The correct position and angle of implant placement in the posterior region is beneficial to the stress distribution of the implant during the function of the implant, and to reduce the risk of bone resorption and abutment, screw, or implant fracture caused by adverse stress. The full-guided template can greatly improve the accuracy of implant placement, and even in the case of insufficient bone conditions, it can also achieve flapless minimally invasive implantation.

In this case, the alveolar crest in the edentulous area has a certain inclination angle, and there is a risk of slipping and deviation when drilling. Using a sharp point drill first to determine the center point of the hole preparation can further improve the accuracy of the hole preparation. In the preparation of pioneer drilling and reaming drilling, it is necessary to start from the shortest 8mm drill, and gradually extend the drill to the required length to ensure that the guide structure of the drill has entered the guide ring when the tip of the drill contacts the alveolar bone, which plays a guiding role. Finally, the Angle errors of implant site 25 and 46 were 1.07° and 1.48°, respectively, and the apical errors were 0.31mm and 0.38mm, respectively, which achieved high accuracy.

In order to ensure the smooth placement of prefabricated immediate interim prosthesis, in addition to accurate implant position and angle, it is also necessary to accurately control the rotation angle of the anti-rotation structure of the implant, which is the rotation angle of the implant along its long axis. This means that the full-guided template must be used. The half-guided template or pioneer-guided template cannot control the rotation angle of the anti-rotation structure of the implant. The current dynamic navigation and implant robot cannot ensure the correct rotation angle of the anti-rotation structure neither. In this case, the accuracy of the implant was placed on the model under the guidance of the full-guided template in the laboratory, and the prefabricated restorations were successfully installed. After verifying the effectiveness of the method, the corresponding surgery and immediate interim restorations were successfully carried out in clinical practice.

本病例通过数字化全程种植导板微创而准确地在左上后牙区及右下后牙区植入两颗种植体，安装预成即刻过渡修复体，并最终将全冠更换为二硅酸锂全冠，恢复患者的咀嚼功能。

In this case, two implants were placed in the left upper posterior area and the right lower posterior area by the digital full-guided template with minimal invasion and maximal accuracy, and the prefabricated immediate interim restorations were installed. Finally, the full lithium disilicate crowns restored the chewing function of the missing teeth.

病例3 数字化全程导板引导上颌中切牙即刻种植并置入术前预成即刻过渡修复体一例

Case 3 Digital Full-guided Template for Immediate Implantation and Immediate Interim Restoration of a Maxillary Central Incisor: A Case Report

本病例资料由闫夏医生、刘海林技师提供，余涛医生整理
Provided from Dr. Xia Yan and Dt. Hailin Liu, and arranged by Dr. Tao Yu

初诊情况

基本信息：30岁女性。

主诉：右上前牙修复体脱落1天。

现病史：1天前，右上前牙修复体脱落，影响美观，无疼痛不适。约10年前上前牙因外伤于外院牙冠修复，之后未出现牙齿疼痛、牙床红肿等不适。否认烟酒嗜好。

既往史：体健。

检查：11四壁缺损均达龈下，叩痛（-），不松动，龈缘略红肿，无溢脓。21全瓷冠修复体完好，叩痛（-），不松动，牙龈无红肿。11龈缘位置较21略偏冠方。11近远中间隙与21近远中径基本一致。前牙覆𬌗覆盖基本正常（图1）。

影像学检查：X线片显示11仅剩余残根，根管内可见根充影响，根尖周未见明显透射影；21根充恰填，根尖周未见明显透射影（图4）。CBCT显示11唇侧牙槽骨壁完整，根方剩余骨量充足，牙槽骨唇舌向宽约8mm（图5）。

Pretreatment

Basic information: 30-year-old female.

Chief complaint: Loss of right upper anterior tooth restoration for 1 day.

History of present illness: One day ago, the restoration of the right upper anterior tooth fell off, affecting the appearance. About 10 years ago, the upper anterior tooth was restored in another hospital due to trauma. Since then, there was no tooth pain, redness and swelling of the gums, or other discomfort occurred. She denied any addictions to tobacco or alcohol.

Past history: In good health.

Examination: For tooth 11, all the four wall defects were subgingival without percussion pain or loose. But the gingival margin was slightly red and swollen. For tooth 21, the all-ceramic crown restoration was in good condition without percussion pain, loosening or any redness and swelling in gingiva. The gingival margin of tooth 11 was slightly more coronal than that of tooth 21. The mesiodistal gap of tooth 11 was approximately the same as the mesiodistal diameter of tooth 21(Fig. 1).

Radiographic examination: Only the residual root of 11 was left with root filling, without obvious radiolucency around the apex. The root canal of 21 was well filled without obvious radiolucency (Fig. 4). 11 had intact alveolar bone wall on the labial side, sufficient residual bone above the apex, and the width of the alveolar bone was about 8mm in the labial and lingual direction (Fig. 5).

诊断

11牙体缺损。

治疗计划

11拔除，即刻种植，植骨，即刻过渡修复，4个月后永久修复。

为了提高种植准确性和尽量减少创伤，计划采用数字化全程导板引导下不翻瓣微创种植。

术前准备

制取口内数字印模，并与术前CBCT一并导入种植导板设计软件（图2和图3），11虚拟设计一颗牙冠，再以修复体为导向设计植入Bredent SKY4.0mm×14mm种植体一颗（图6和图7），完成全程种植导板设计并输出虚拟设计的种植体位置，依照此位置设计即刻过渡修复体的个性化基台和外冠。3D打印种植导板并粘接金属导环（图8），在模型上试戴导板，贴合、稳定、固位力良好（图9）。切削Bio-HPP个性化基台和复合树脂外冠（图10）。考虑到即刻种植后软硬组织改建过程中可能出现的龈缘退缩风险，而治疗前的龈缘较对侧略偏冠方，因此按照治疗前龈缘位置制作过渡修复体，保存更多的软组织高度，使之在种植位点完全愈合后具备更多可塑形潜力（图11）。为了术中即刻过渡修复体戴牙更顺利，制作硅橡胶戴牙导板（图12）。

Diagnosis

11 tooth defect.

Treatment plan

11 Extraction, immediate implant, bone graft, immediate interim restoration, and permanent restoration after 4 months.

In order to improve the accuracy of implantation and minimize trauma, the digital full-guided template was planned to be used for flapless minimally invasive implantation.

Preoperative preparation

The intraoral digital impression was taken and imported into the implant guide design software together with the preoperative CBCT (Figs. 2 and 3). A crown was virtually designed, and then a Bredent SKY 4.0×14mm implant was planned according to prosthodontic-oriented design (Figs. 6 and 7). The whole process of implant guide template design was completed, and the implant position of the virtual design was output. According to this position, the personalized abutment and crown of the immediate interim restoration were designed. The 3D printed implant guide template and metal guide ring were bonded (Fig. 8). When the guide template was seated on the model, it showed good fit, stability, and retention (Fig. 9). Bio-HPP personalized abutment and composite resin outer crown were milled (Fig. 10). Considering the possible risk of gingival margin recession during the reconstruction of soft and hard tissues after immediate implantation, the pre-treatment gingival margin was slightly more coronal than the contralateral side. Therefore, the interim restoration was fabricated according to the pre-treatment gingival margin position to preserve more soft tissue height and had more shaping potential after the healing of the implant site (Fig. 11). To ensure a smoother wearing of the interim restoration during the procedure, a silicone rubber guide template was fabricated. (Fig. 12).

1 ~ 7 术前检查与导板设计
Preoperative examination and the design of the
surgical template

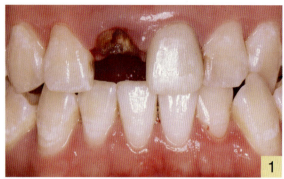

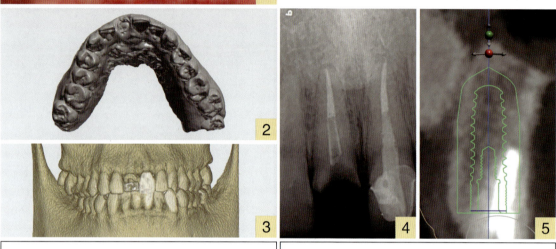

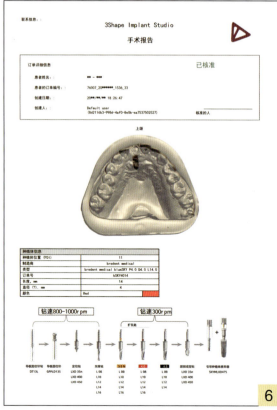

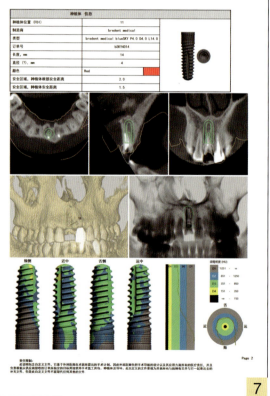

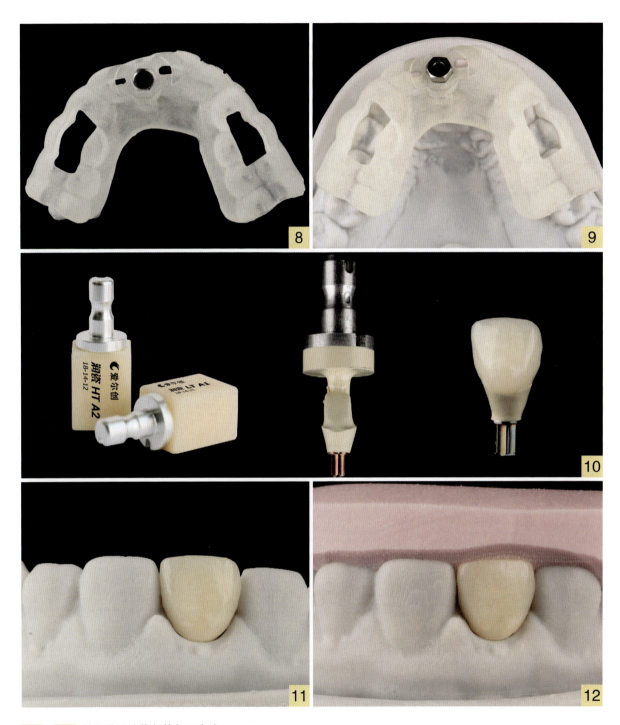

8 ~ 12 导板及过渡修复体加工完成
The fabrication of the surgical template and the interim restoration

治疗过程

常规消毒铺巾后，11局部浸润麻醉，微创拔牙器械拔除患牙，牙根完整，搔刮并冲洗拔牙窝，探查骨壁完整（图13~图17）。确认导板完全就位后贴合、稳定、固位良好，导板引导下定点，逐级备洞，使用引导型种植体携带器植入Bredent SKY4.0mm×14mm、种植体一颗，直至携带器止动环与导环贴合，二者六边形结构完全重叠，植入扭矩大于45Ncm（图18~图20）。取下引导型种植体携带器，再取下导板，见种植体位置良好（图21），双区植骨，严密植入低替代率骨代用品（图22）。安装术前制作的个性化Bio-HPP基台，旋紧螺丝至25Ncm，暂封螺丝孔，试戴复合树脂外冠，临时粘接剂粘接，确保该修复体无咬合接触（图23~图28）。

术后验证种植准确度，11种植体植入角度误差0.71°，根尖区误差0.49mm（图29）。

4个月后，11修复体完好，不松动，种植体不松动，牙龈无红肿，龈缘位置较对侧略偏冠方。为了获取更加对称的牙龈形态，11重新制作了过渡修复体，将龈缘塑形至左右基本对称的状态（图30~图36）。牙龈成熟后左右对称，由于过渡修复体形态未做任何改变，因此永久修复体可以使用该过渡修复体的设计数据，更换永久修复体材料制作即可，无需再次制取印模。试戴永久修复体，个性化Bio-HPP基台就位后上紧至25Ncm，树脂封闭螺丝孔，树脂水门汀粘接全瓷外冠，拍摄X线片显示修复体完全就位，全瓷冠边缘密合，无粘接剂

Treatment process

After routine disinfection and local anesthesia, minimally invasive extraction instruments were used to extract the residual root of tooth 11. The root had no cracks, and the bone of the socket was detected to be intact (Figs. 13 to 17). After making sure that the guide template was fitted, stable and well retained, the holes were prepared step by step under the guidance of the guide template. Then the guided implant carrier was screwed onto one Bredent SKY 4.0×14mm implant. The implant was inserted to the bone until the stop ring contacted the guide ring and the hexagonal structure of the two rings completely overlapped. The insertion torque is greater than 45Ncm (Figs. 18 to 20). The guided implant carrier was removed, and then the guided template was removed to see that the implant was in good position (Fig. 21). Low replacement rate bone substitute was tightly implanted (Fig. 22). The personalized Bio-HPP abutment fabricated before operation was installed. The screws were tightened to 25Ncm and the screw holes were temporarily sealed. The composite resin crown was fitted, and the temporary adhesive was applied. The restoration had no occlusal contact (Figs. 23 to 28).

The accuracy of implant placement was verified after operation. The angle error of 11 implant was 0.71°, and the error in the apical area was 0.49mm (Fig. 29).

Four months later, the restoration and the implant were intact and stable, the gingiva was not red or swollen, and the position of the gingival margin was slightly more coronal than the contralateral side. To obtain a more symmetrical gingival shape, another interim restoration was delivered to shape the gingival margin (Figs. 30 to 36). The gingival margins of both central incisors were symmetrical after shaping, with no adjustments needed for the interim restoration. Consequently, there was no requirement to take an impression for the definitive restoration, which can be fabricated using the homologous design data from the interim restoration, only changing the materials to definitive ones. The customized Bio-HPP abutment was tightened to 25Ncm, the screw holes were closed with resin, and the all-ceramic crown was bonded with

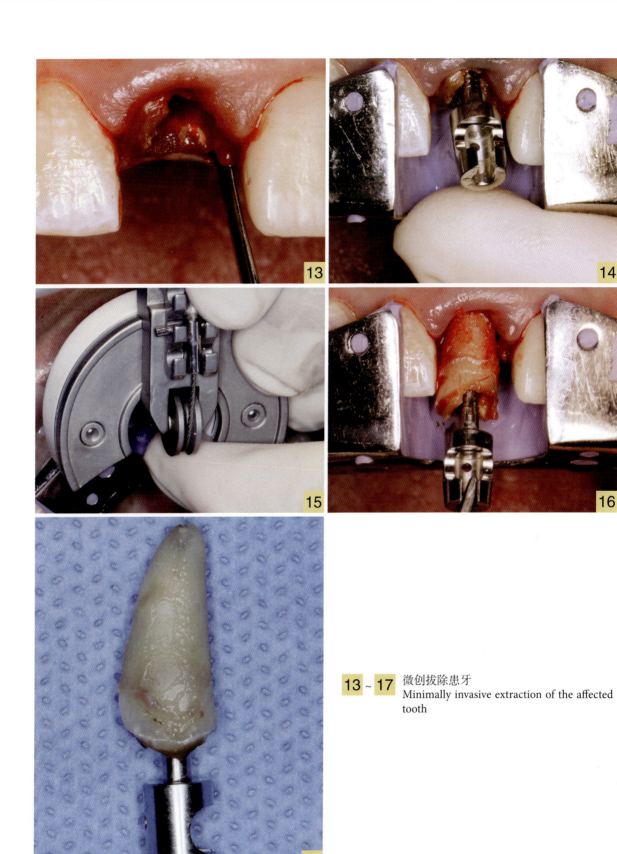

13 ~ 17 微创拔除患牙
Minimally invasive extraction of the affected tooth

残留。11种植体周围软组织无红肿，双侧龈缘高度基本对称，软组织丰满度足够，牙冠形态、颜色自然，最终修复效果满意（图37～图42）。

resin cement. The periapical X-ray film showed that the prosthesis was fully in place, the edge of the all-ceramic crown was fit, and no adhesive remained. There was no redness and swelling of the soft tissue around the implant. The height of the bilateral gingival margin was basically symmetrical. The fullness of the soft tissue was desirable. The shape and color of the crown were natural. And the final restoration effect was satisfactory (Figs. 37 to 42).

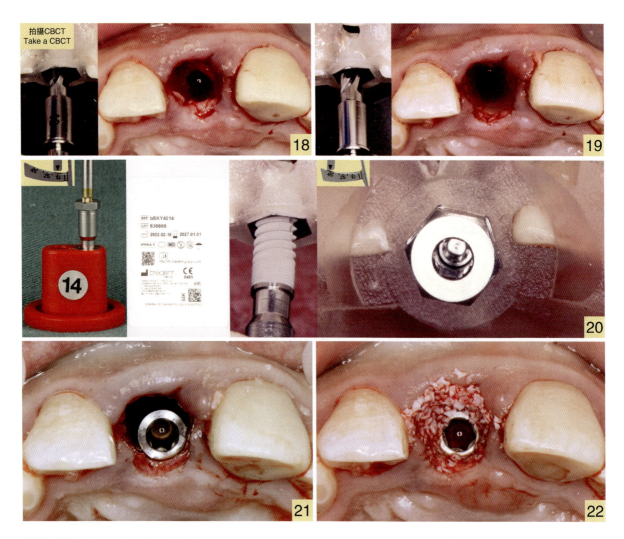

18～22 导板引导下植入种植体
Implant placement with the surgical template

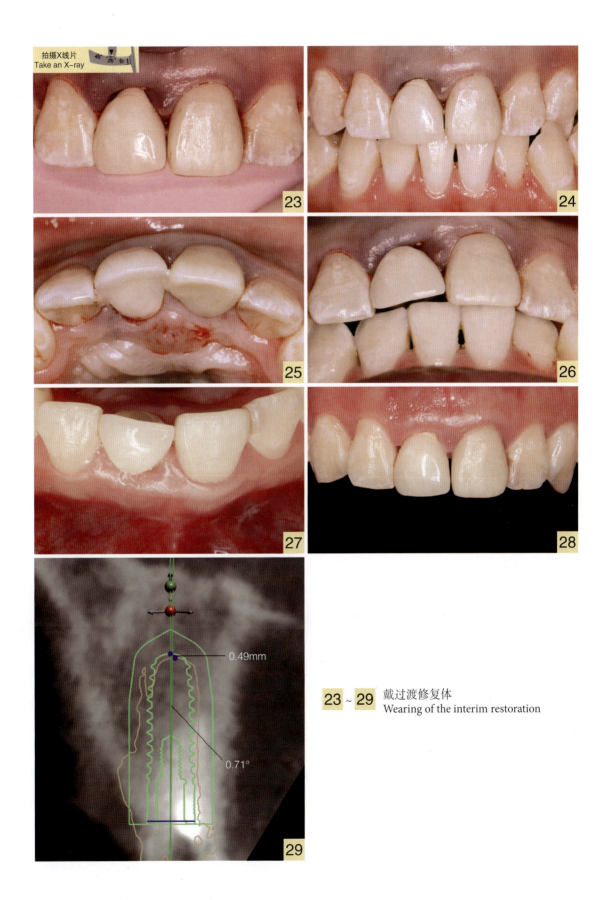

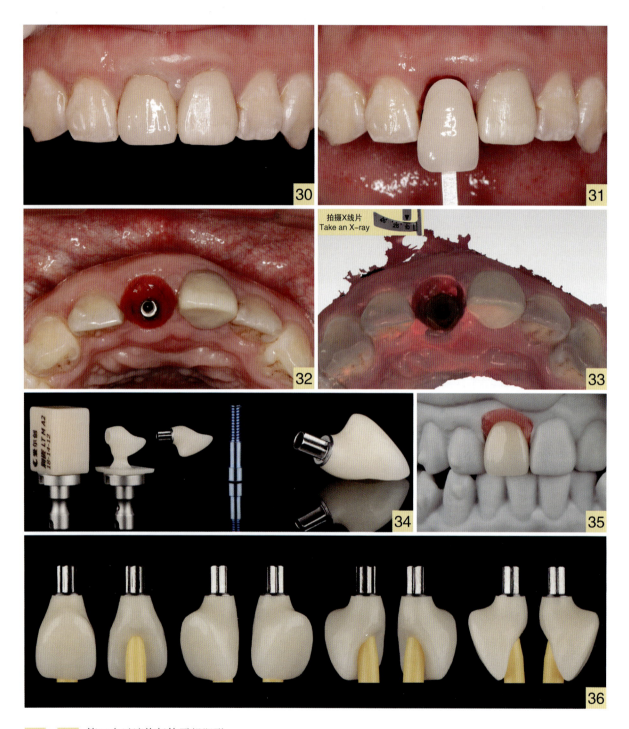

30 ~ 36 第二个过渡修复体牙龈塑形
A second interim restoration to shape the gingiva

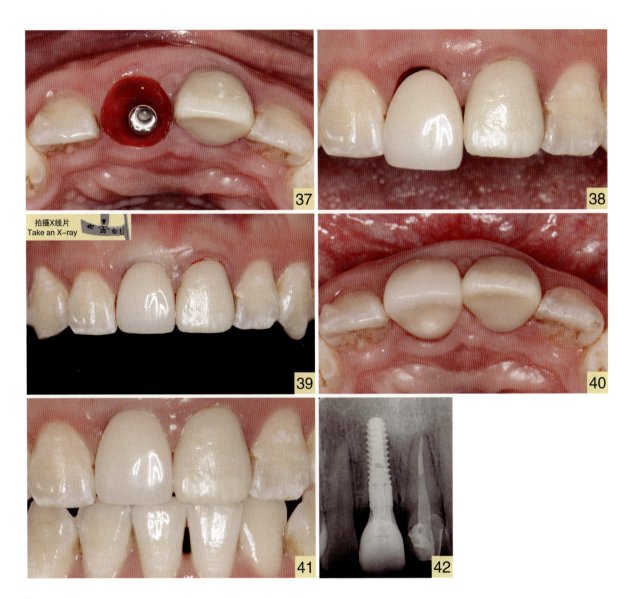

37 ~ 42　戴永久修复体
Wearing of the definitive restoration

讨论

上前牙区种植修复是美学要求最高的区域，需要将种植体植入正确的位置与轴向。受牙槽骨密度不均匀带来的侧向力影响，种植体容易偏唇侧，导致牙龈退缩，美学效果不佳。尤其是上前牙区即刻种植备洞和种植体植入时，一般腭侧阻力较大而唇侧阻力小，钻针和种植体受到较大的侧向力，容易偏唇侧。种植导板能够很好地约束钻针和种植体携带器，有效降低侧向力对种植体植入准确度的影响。本病例11种植位点的植入角度误差仅0.71°，根尖误差0.49mm°，准确度较高。

即刻种植、跳跃间隙植骨、即刻修复有利于保存种植体唇侧牙槽骨高度，同时简化治疗程序，缩短治疗周期。本病例在即刻过渡修复体设计时，也为软组织生长保留了略多余对侧的空间，以保证获得足够的软组织量，便于后期软组织塑形。当种植位点愈合之后，制作第二个过渡修复体，将牙龈塑形至左右基本对称，达到满意的美观效果。永久修复体使用了与过渡修复体同源数据，非常完美且简便地复制穿龈轮廓。

本病例通过数字化全程种植导板微创而准确地完成右上中切牙即刻种植，并安装预成即刻过渡修复体，并通过第二个过渡修复体塑形，使用口内数字印模准确复制其穿龈轮廓，制作的最终修复体获得了较为满意的美学效果。

Discussion

The upper anterior region is the most aesthetically demanding area, necessitating precise implant placement in terms of position and direction. Due to the lateral forces resulting from uneven alveolar bone density, implants are prone to tilting toward the labial side, causing gingival recession and suboptimal aesthetic outcomes. This issue is particularly pronounced in immediate implant placement procedures in the maxillary anterior region, where the resistance on the palatal side is significantly higher than on the labial side, making drills and implants susceptible to labial tilting under large lateral forces. The use of a guided surgical template can effectively stabilize the drills and implant carrier, thereby mitigating the impact of lateral forces on placement accuracy. In this case, the angle error of the implant placement was only 0.71°, and the apical error was 0.49mm, demonstrating high precision.

Immediate implant placement, bone grafting, and immediate restoration can help preserve the height of the labial alveolar bone of the implant, simplify the treatment procedure, and shorten the treatment period. In this case, the design of the immediate interim restoration reserved slightly more space for the growth of soft tissue to ensure that enough soft tissue was obtained for later shaping. After the implant site healed, the second interim restoration was fabricated to shape the gingiva to create symmetric gingival margins to achieve a satisfactory aesthetic effect. The emergence profile was perfectly and easily replicated using homologous data from the interim restoration when fabricating the definitive restoration.

In this case, the digital full-guided implant template was used to place an implant for the right upper central incisor immediately with minimal invasion and high accuracy, and the prefabricated interim restoration was installed. The intraoral digital impression was used to accurately reproduce the emergence profile of the interim restoration.

病例4 终末期牙列数字化全程导板全口种植即刻修复一例

Case 4 Immediate Implant-supported Restorations with Digital Full-guided Templates for Terminal Dentitions: A Case Report

本病例资料由Arnulf-Reimar Metzmacher医生、刘海林技师提供，余涛医生整理

Provided from Dr. Arnulf-Reimar Metzmacher and Dt. Hailin Liu, and arranged by Dr. Tao Yu

初诊情况

基本信息：65岁女性。

主诉：双侧上下颌前后牙缺失10余年。

现病史：10余年以来，上下颌多颗前后牙缺失，未曾修复，诉咀嚼无力，近期又有牙齿缺失、缺损，剩余多颗牙齿松动，咀嚼功能低下，现咨询种植固定修复。

既往史：糖尿病，服药控制空腹血糖约7mmol/L。

检查：17-14、23-27、37、31、41、46、47缺失，牙槽骨中度至重度吸收。12-22、32、42、36过长，松动Ⅱ～Ⅲ度，牙龈退缩。13、33、43松动Ⅰ度。34、35、44、45松动Ⅰ度。高位笑线，微笑时上前牙区牙龈暴露3～4mm（图1～图5）。

影像学检查：CBCT显示余留牙牙槽骨普遍吸收至根尖1/3或超过根尖；双侧上颌前磨牙区及前牙区、下颌颏孔之间骨量尚可。

Pretreatment

Basic information: 65-year-old woman.

Chief complaint: Bilateral anterior and posterior teeth missing for more than 10 years.

History of present illness: The patient had multiple anterior and posterior teeth missing for more than 10 years without restoration, complaining of masticatory weakness. Recently, the patient had tooth loss and defect, and the remaining teeth were loose, and the chewing function was low.

Past history: Diabetes mellitus, taking medicine to control fasting blood glucose about 7mmol/L.

Examination: 17-14, 23-27, 37, 31, 41, 46, 47 were missing with moderate to severe alveolar resorption. 12-22, 32, 42, 36 were too long with II to III° mobility. 13, 33, 43, 34, 35, 44, 45 had I° mobility. High smile line showed 3 to 4mm gingival exposure in the upper anterior area when smiling (Figs. 1 to 5).

Radiographic examination: CBCT showed that the alveolar bone of the residual teeth was generally absorbed to the apical third or beyond the apical third. The bone mass of bilateral maxillary premolar area, anterior teeth area, and mandibular mental foraminal area was acceptable .

诊断

1. 上下颌牙列缺损。
2. 慢性牙周炎。

治疗计划

拔除所有余留牙，即刻上下颌All-on-4种植，即刻过渡修复，4个月后永久修复。

术前准备

由于患者上颌后牙已经全部缺失，目前缺乏稳定的咬合支持；因此先为患者制作了上颌放射导板，确定颌位关系，并佩戴放射导板再次进行CBCT扫描。将放射导板进行光学扫描，作为制作上颌导板的数字模型，与下颌口扫、CBCT一并导入导板设计软件。

分别于15、25、35、45位点设计斜行植入Bredent SKY 4.5mm×14mm种植体各一颗，于12、22位点设计直立植入Bredent SKY 3.5mm×14mm种植体各一颗，于32、42位点直立植入Bredent SKY 4.0mm×14mm种植体各一颗。上颌余留牙无法为导板提供稳定的支持，因此上颌设计为黏膜支持式导板，放置4颗固位针；下颌34、35、44、45牙齿并不妨碍种植体植入位置，且这些牙齿较为稳定，可以为导板提供稳定支持，因此下颌设计为混合支持式导板，放置3颗固位针（图6和图7）。15、25两颗种植体颈部向远中倾斜，避免损伤上颌窦，同时尽量使复合基台穿出位置偏向远中，

Diagnosis

1. Maxillary and mandibular dentition defect.
2. Chronic periodontitis.

Treatment plan

All remaining teeth were planned to be extracted, and immediate All-on-4 implants were planned to be placed in the upper and lower jaws with immediate interim restoration and definitive restoration after 4 months.

Preoperative preparation

Because the patient's maxillary posterior teeth have all been missing, there is currently a lack of stable occlusal support. Therefore, the maxillary radiation guided template was made for the patient to determine the jaw relationship, and the patient wore the radiation guided template for CBCT scanning again. The optical scanning of the guided template was used as the digital model of the maxillary guided template, which was imported into the guide design software together with the mandibular oral scan and CBCT.

One Bredent SKY 4.5×14mm implant was designed to be placed oblique at 15, 25, 35, and 45 sites respectively, and one Bredent SKY 3.5×14mm implant was designed to be placed upright at 12 and 22 sites respectively. One Bredent SKY 4.0×14mm implant was placed upright at sites 32 and 42. The maxillary residual teeth could not provide stable support for the guided template. Therefore, the maxillary mucosa support guided template was designed, and 4 fixation pins were placed. The mandibular teeth 34, 35, 44, and 45 did not interfere with the position of implant placement, and these teeth were relatively stable and could provide stable support for the guided template. Therefore, the mandibular was designed as a mixed-support guided template, and three retention needles were placed (Figs. 6 and 7). The two implants of 15 and 25 were tilted distally to avoid damage to the maxillary sinus. At the same time, the multi-unit abutments were tilted distally to minimize the length of the distal cantilever (Figs. 12 and 14). The two implants of 12 and 22 were positioned below the crest of

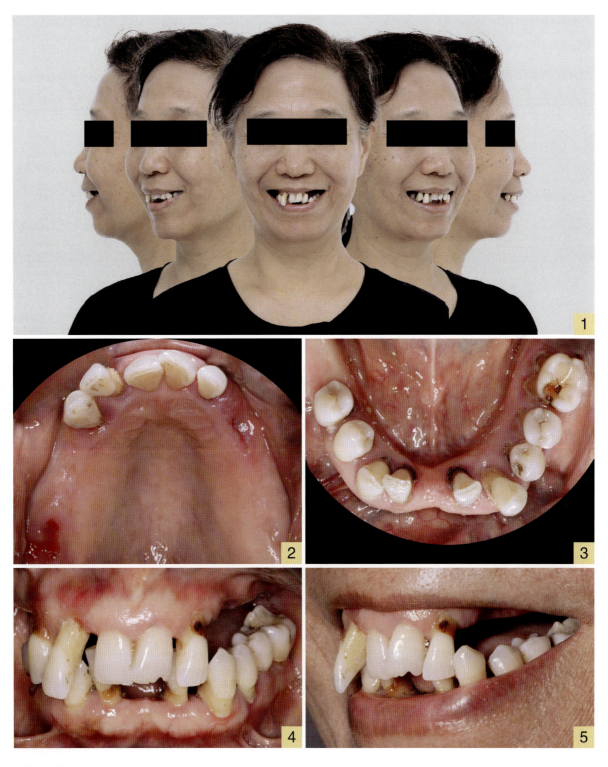

1 ~ 5 术前检查
Pretreatment examination

减小远中悬臂长度（图12和图14）。12、22两颗种植体颈部位于牙槽嵴顶以下，保证足够的修复空间，并便于上颌前部牙槽骨修整，以避免修复完成后微笑时暴露义齿-黏膜界面（图11和图13）。35、45两颗种植体颈部向远中倾斜，避免损伤颏孔及下牙槽神经管，同时尽量使复合基台穿出位置偏向远中，减小远中悬臂长度（图16和图18）。32、42两颗种植体颈部位于牙槽嵴顶以下，保证足够的修复空间，并与远中两颗种植体颈部高度基本持平（图15和图17）。完成导板设计后，3D打印导板，粘接相应金属导环，准备导板手术工具盒（图8~图10）。

治疗过程

常规消毒铺巾后，16-26局部浸润麻醉，13-22微创拔除，牙根完整，牙槽窝搔刮并用3%H_2O_2与生理盐水冲洗，探查骨壁完整无折断（图19）。上颌导板就位后稳定，使用固位针钻备洞，并安装4颗固位针固定上颌导板（图25、图26和图20）。依次使用定位钻、先锋钻、扩孔钻、颈部成型钻逐级备洞（图27~图30）。取出种植体并安装引导型种植体携带器，旋紧螺丝至10Ncm，导板引导下植入种植体，直至携带器止动环与导环完全贴合，植入扭矩均不低于45Ncm（图21、图31~图34）。安装Fast-Fix复合基台，穿出位置基本位于未来修复体牙冠殆面，上紧扭矩至25Ncm（图22和图23）。每个复合基台上安装复合基台保护帽，旋紧扭矩10Ncm（图24），上颌手术完成。

the alveolar ridge to ensure adequate restoration space and facilitate the shaping of the alveolar bone in the anterior maxillary region to avoid exposing the denture-mucosa interface during smile after restoration delivery (Figs. 11 and 13). The two implants of 35 and 45 were tilted distally to avoid any damage to the bilateral mental foramen and inferior alveolar nerve canals. At the same time, the multi-unit abutments were tilted to the distally and the length of the distal cantilever was reduced as far as possible (Figs. 16 and 18). The two implants of 32 and 42 was positioned below the crest of the alveolar ridge to ensure adequate restoration space and was basically at the same height as the neck of the two distal implants (Figs. 15 and 17). After the design of the guided template was completed, the guided template was 3D printed, the corresponding metal guide ring was bonded, and the surgical toolbox of the guided template was prepared (Figs. 8 to 10).

Treatment process

After routine disinfection and drape, 16-26 local infiltration anesthesia, 13-22 minimally invasive extraction, intact root, alveolar fossa curettage and irrigation with 3%H_2O_2 and saline, and intact bone wall detected without fracture (Fig. 19). After the maxillary guided template was stabilized in place, holes were drilled using a fixation pin drill, and 4 pins were installed to fix the maxillary guided template (Figs. 25, 26, and 20). Position drill, pioneer drill, reaming drill, and neck molding drill were used to prepare the hole step by step in turn (Figs. 27 to 30). The implant were removed and the guided implant carrier was installed. The screws were tightened with 10Ncm, and the implants were placed under the guidance of the guided template until the stop ring of the carrier was completely fitted to the guide ring. The insertion torque was not lower than 45Ncm (Figs. 21, 31 to 34). The fast-fix multi-unit abutment was installed, and the piercing position was located at the occlusal surface of the crown of the future restoration, and the tightening torque was 25Ncm (Figs. 22 and 23). The multi-unit abutment protective cap was installed on each multi-unit abutment with a tightening torque of 10Ncm (Fig. 24), and the maxillary surgery was completed.

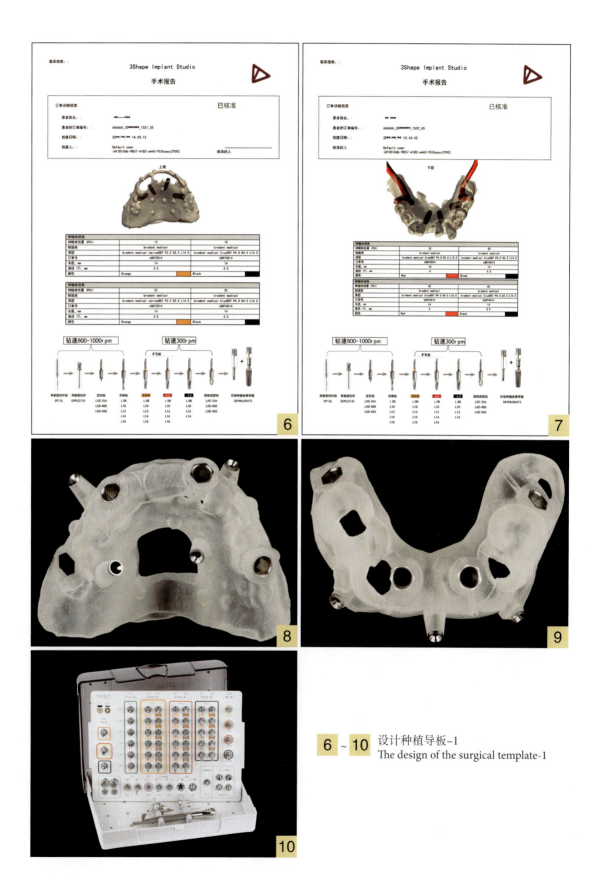

6 ~ 10 设计种植导板–1
The design of the surgical template-1

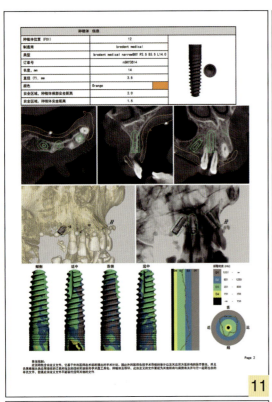

11

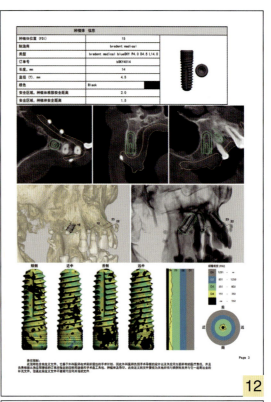

12

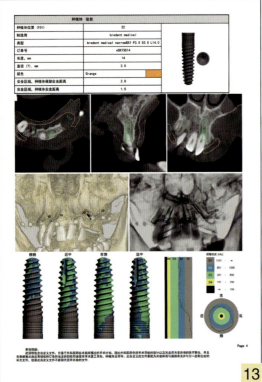

13

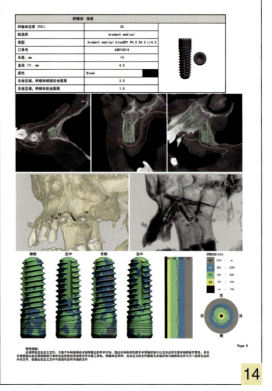

14

11 ~ 14 设计种植导板–2
The design of the surgical template-2

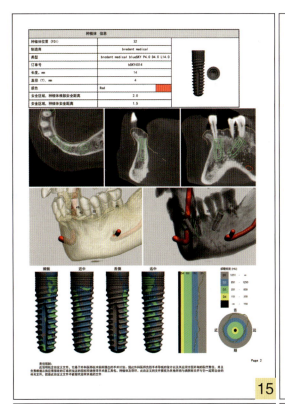

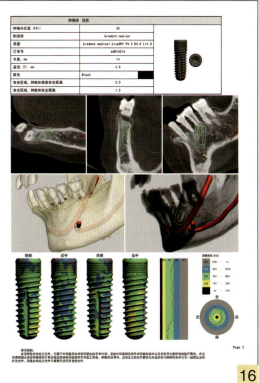

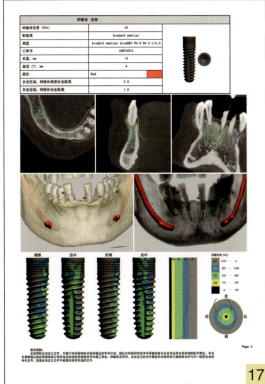

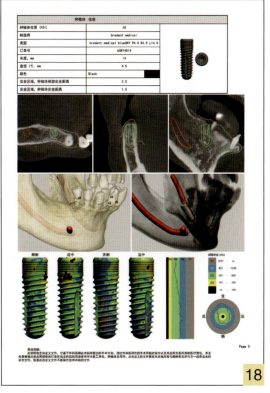

15 ~ 18 设计种植导板-3
The design of the surgical template-3

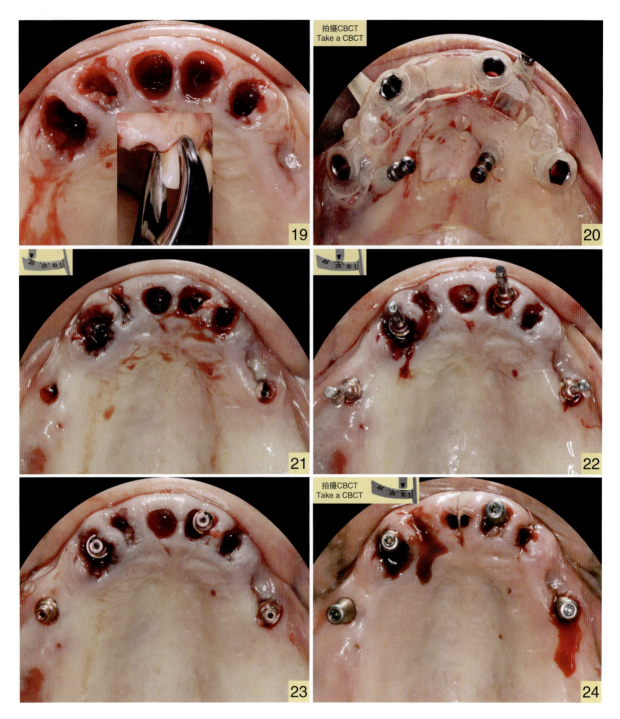

19 ~ 24 上颌术中概览
Overview of the surgery of the maxilla

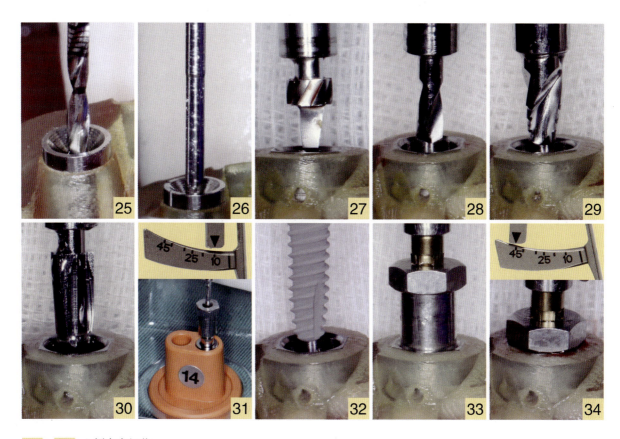

25～34 上颌术中细节
Details of the surgery of the maxilla

36-46局部浸润麻醉，36、33、32、42、43微创拔除，牙根完整，牙槽窝搔刮并用3%H$_2$O$_2$与生理盐水冲洗，探查骨壁完整无折断（图35和图41），暂时保留34、35、44、45。下颌导板就位后稳定，使用固位针钻备洞，并安装3颗固位针固定下颌导板（图42、图43和图36）。依次使用定位钻、先锋钻、扩孔钻、颈部成型钻逐级备洞（图44～图48）。取出种植体并安装引导型种植体携带器，旋紧螺丝至10Ncm，导板引导下33、42位点植入种植体，直至携带器止动环与导环完全贴合，植入扭矩均不低于

Local infiltration anesthesia was taken between 36 to 46. Then 36, 33, 32, 42, 43 were minimally invasive extraction. The alveolar bone was scratched, irrigated, and probed to be intact without fracture (Figs. 35 and 41). 34, 35, 44, 45 were temporarily remained. After the mandibular guided template was in place and stabilized, holes were prepared using a drill of fixation pin, and 3 fixation pins were installed to fix the mandibular guided template (Figs. 42, 43, and 36). The positioning drill, pioneer drill, reaming drill, and neck molding drill were used to prepare the hole step by step in turn (Figs. 44 to 48). The implant was removed and the guided implant carrier was installed. The screws were tightened to 10Ncm, and for site 33 and 42, the implants were placed under the guidance of the guided template until the stop

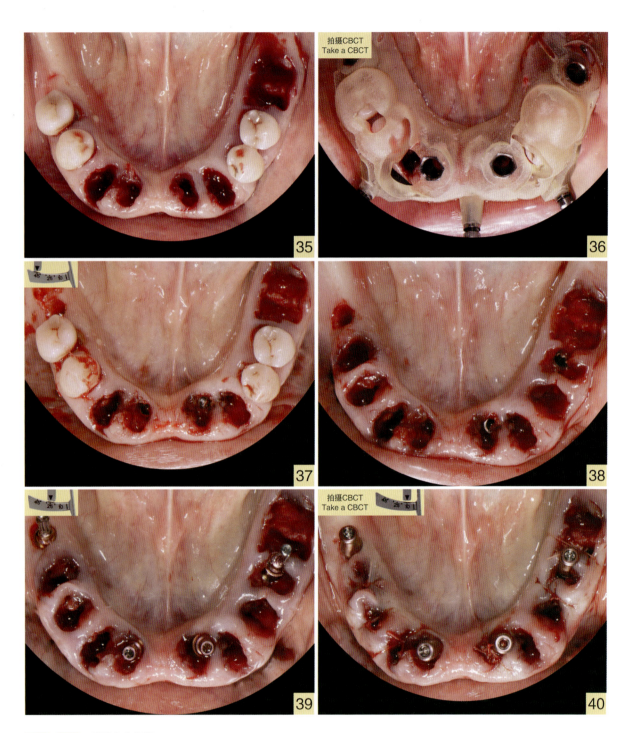

35 ~ 40 下颌术中概览
Overview of the surgery of the mandibular

45Ncm（图49和图50），取下导板（图37），微创拔除34、35、44、45，于36、46位点植入种植体（图38、图51~图53），安装Fast-Fix复合基台，穿出位置基本位于未来修复体牙冠殆面，上紧扭矩至25Ncm（图39）。每个复合基台上安装复合基台保护帽，旋紧扭矩10Ncm（图40），下颌手术完成。

拍片确认所有种植体位置良好，复合基台完全就位后，取下复合基台保护帽，安装复合基台水平转移杆，使用牙科种植用连接件+成型树脂在口内连接，上下颌均使用硅橡胶制取开窗夹板式基台水平印模。再次安装复合基台保护帽，硅橡胶制取颌位记录，确定中线、殆平面。转技工室灌模型，上殆架，制作即刻过渡义齿。并于手术当天取下复合基台保护帽，为患者戴入即刻过渡义齿（图56），拍片确认义齿完全就位（图55）。由于不翻瓣手术创伤较小，导板手术术中时间较短，手术当天就初步恢复患者的咀嚼功能并极大改善美观效果，患者对手术过程及义齿较为满意（图54）。

ring of the carrier was completely fitted to the guide ring, and the insertion torque was not lower than 45Ncm for each implant (Figs. 49 and 50). The guided template was removed (Fig. 37). For site 36 and 46, the implants were inserted after minimally invasive extraction of 34, 35, 44, 45 (Figs. 38, 51 to 53). A torque of 25Ncm was applied to install the fast-fix multi-unit abutments of whom the secondary screw holes passed through the occlusal surface of the future restoration (Fig. 39). Multi-unit abutment protective caps were installed on each multi-unit abutment with a tightening torque of 10Ncm (Fig. 40), and the mandibular surgery was completed.

After the multi-unit abutments were completely in place, the protective cap was removed, the transfer copings of the multi-unit abutment were installed, and the steel pod and pattern resin were used to connect the transfer copings. The impressions were made with silicone rubber. The multi-unit abutment protective caps were installed again, and the maxilla-mandible position was recorded by silicone rubber to determine the midline and occlusal plane. The casts were irrigated in the lab, and the casts were put on the articulator to produce the immediate transition restorations. On the day of surgery, the protective caps of the multi-unit abutment were removed, and the immediate transition restorations were placed in the patient's mouth (Fig. 56). X-ray film was taken to confirm that the restorations were completely in place (Fig. 55). Due to the less trauma of the flapless surgery and the shorter intraoperative time of the template surgery, the masticatory function of the patients was initially restored and the aesthetic effect was greatly improved on the day of surgery. The patient was satisfied with the operation process and restorations (Fig. 54).

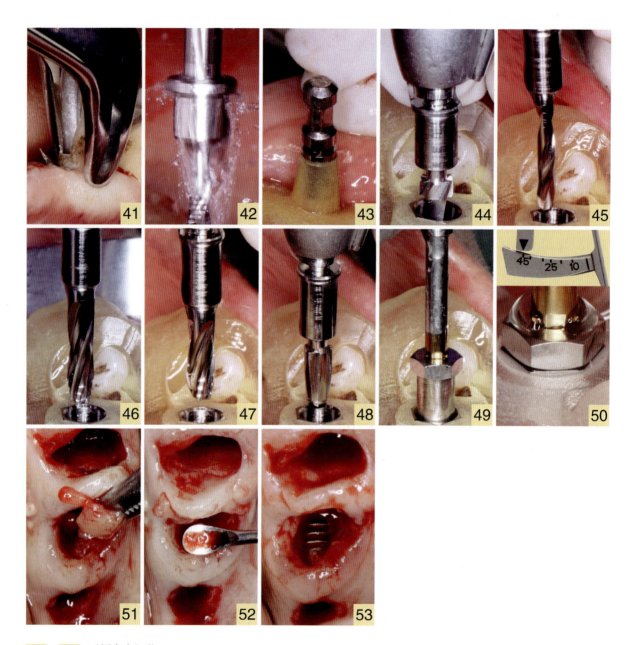

41 ~ 53 下颌术中细节
Details of the surgery of the mandibular

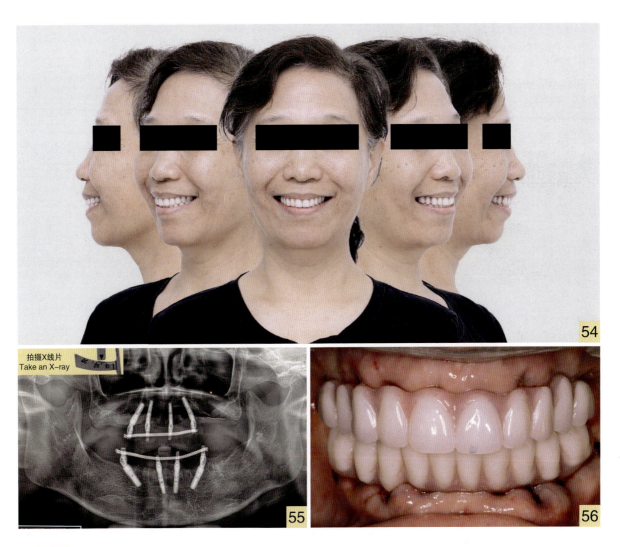

拍摄X线片
Take an X-ray

54 ~ 56 戴即刻过渡义齿
Delivery of the immediate restorations

过渡修复4个月后，患者无不适主诉，义齿稳定，种植体无松动，周围无明显炎症。将所有复合基台再次加力至25Ncm，安装复合基台转移杆并用成型树脂于口内再次连接，使用个别托盘制取上下颌硅橡胶开窗夹板式基台水平印模，灌制石膏模型，用过渡义齿与硅橡胶

After 4 months of interim restoration, the patient had no complaints of discomfort, the restorations were stable, and there was no loosening of the implant and no obvious inflammation around the implant. All the multi-unit abutments were re-forced to 25Ncm, and the multi-unit abutment transfer copings were installed and re-connected with pattern resin in the mouth. The impressions of the upper and lower jaw were made by using individual trays, and the plaster casts were filled.

制取咬合记录并将模型上𬌗架。为患者制作评估桥（图59），戴入口内后拍片确认完全就位（图58），评估桥中线、𬌗平面正确，前牙丰满度合适，垂直距离合适，正中关系正确，双侧咬合均匀稳定，患者对牙齿排列满意（图57）。

数字化复制评估桥外形，并回切全瓷牙冠及牙龈部分烤塑空间（图60和图61）。切削PMMA支架，验证回切空间合适（图62、图63和图66）。切削正式钛架，并确认全瓷牙冠修复及牙龈部分烤塑空间合适（图64、图65和图67）。钛架表面遮色，光学扫描，设计16-26、36-46全瓷冠，并用高透渐变色氧化锆制作全锆冠，仅进行外染色而不加饰瓷。牙龈部分进行烤塑，模拟天然牙龈颜色。染色上釉后的义齿再上𬌗架调𬌗，正中𬌗双侧后牙均匀接触，前伸𬌗多颗前牙均匀接触而后牙脱离接触，侧方𬌗工作侧为组牙功能𬌗（图68～图75）。再将义齿进行最终抛光，完成制作（图76～图80）。

将义齿于患者口内试戴，上紧二级螺丝至18Ncm，并拍摄X线片确定义齿完全就位（图82）。使用聚四氟乙烯膜+流动树脂封闭螺丝孔，在患者口内调𬌗，抛光，完成义齿修复（图83～图85）。患者获得了良好的咀嚼功能和美观效果（图81），其笑容较治疗前有明显改善（图86～图89）。

Evaluation bridges were made for the patient (Fig. 59), and an X-ray was taken to confirm that they was completely in place (Fig. 58). It was evaluated that the middle line and occlusal plane of the bridge were correct, the fullness of the anterior teeth was appropriate, the vertical distance was appropriate, the centric relationship was correct, the bilateral occlusion was uniform and stable, and the patient was satisfied with the arrangement of the teeth (Fig. 57).

The shapes of the bridges were evaluated by digital copy, and the plastic space of the full porcelain crown and the gingiva was cut back (Figs. 60 and 61). The PMMA frameworks were cut to verify that the backcut space was suitable (Figs. 62, 63, and 66). Cut the formal titanium frameworks and confirm that the full ceramic crown restoration and gum part baking plastic space were appropriate (Figs. 64, 65, and 67). The surface of the titanium frameworks was opaque, optical scanned. 16-26, 36-46 all-ceramic crowns were designed, and the high-transparence gradient zirconia was used to make all-zirconium crowns. Only external staining was performed without porcelain decoration. The gingival part was baked and molded to simulate the natural gingival color. After dyeing and glaze, the restorations were put on the articulator to adjust the occlusion. The posterior teeth on both sides were evenly contacted in centric occlusion. The multiple anterior teeth were evenly contacted in protrusive occlusion and the posterior teeth were out of contact. The working side of the lateral occlusion was group functional occlusion (Figs. 68 to 75). The final polishing of the denture was carried out to complete the production (Figs. 76 to 80).

The restorations were tried in the patient's mouth. The secondary screws were tightened to 18Ncm. An X-ray was taken to confirm that the restorations were fully in place (Fig. 82). The screw holes were closed with PTFE membrane + flowable resin. adjustment and polishing were carried out in the patient's mouth to complete the restorations (Figs. 83 to 85). The patient obtained good masticatory function and aesthetic results (Fig. 81), and the smile was significantly improved compared with that before treatment (Figs. 86 to 89).

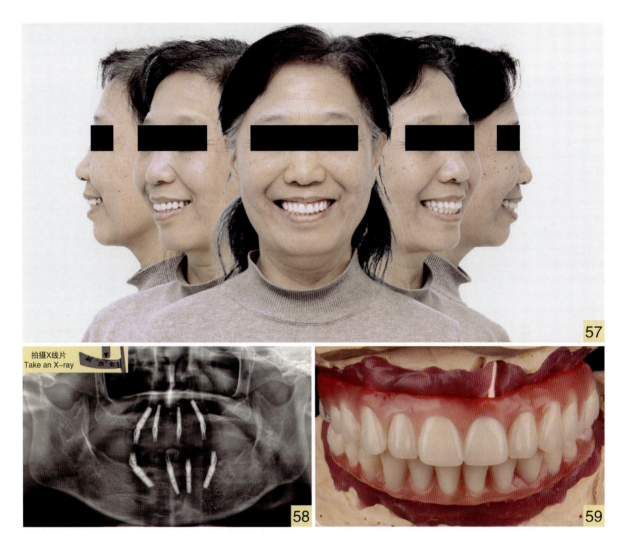

拍摄X线片
Take an X-ray

57 ~ 59 试戴评估桥
Try-in of evaluation bridge

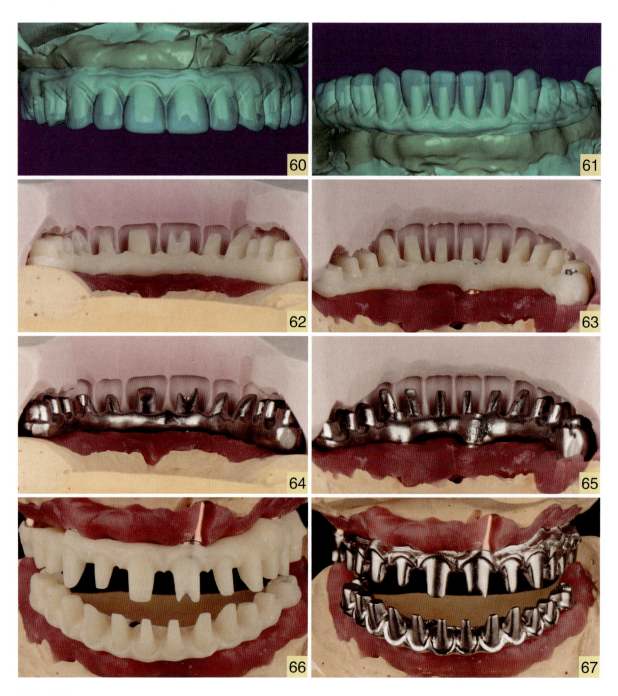

60 ~ 67　制作钛桥架
Machined titanium frameworks

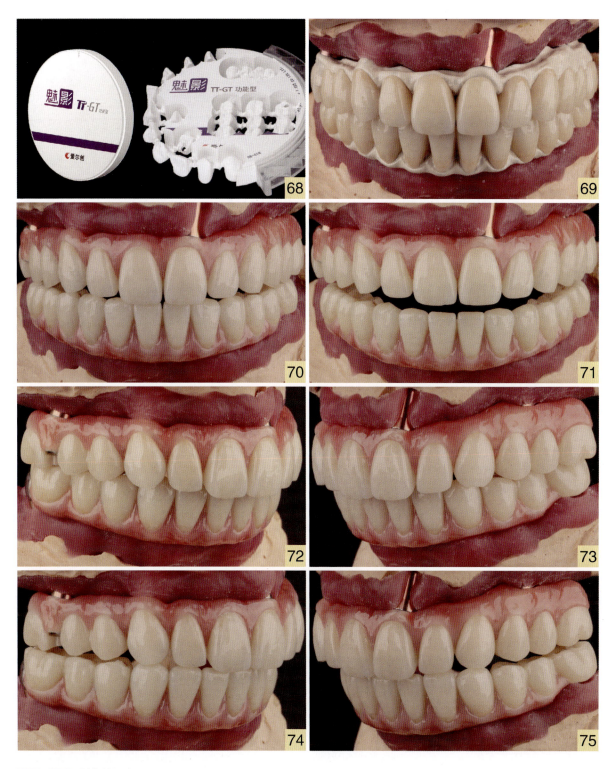

68 ~ 75　制作外冠
Fabricating zirconia crowns

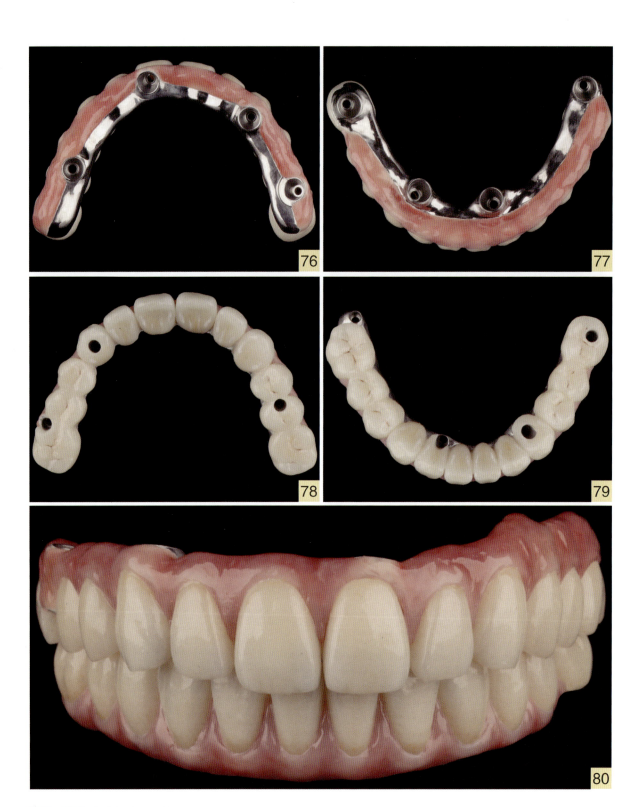

76 ~ 80 完成的永久义齿
Finished definitive restorations

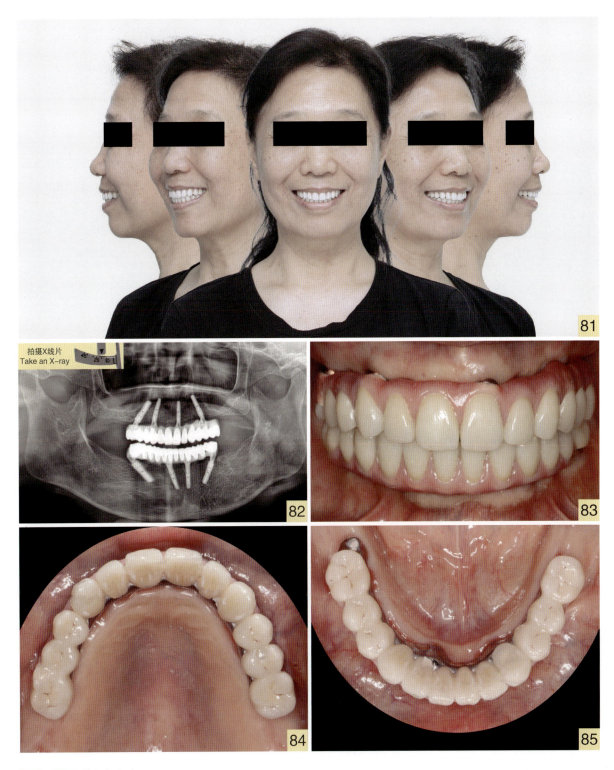

81 ~ 85 戴永久义齿
Delivery of the definitive restorations

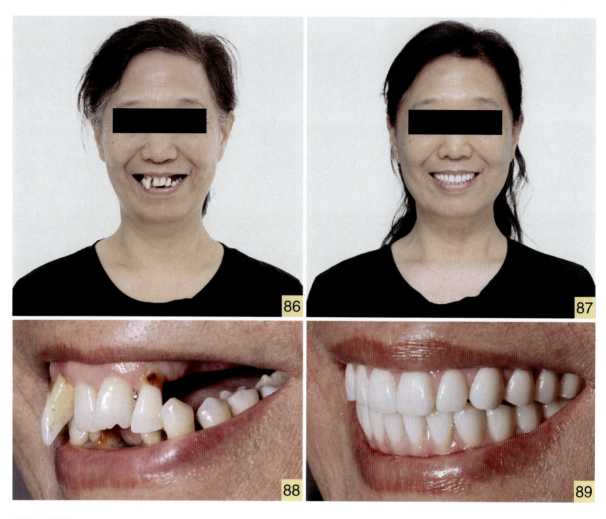

86 ~ 89 术前术后对比
Comparation of pre- and post-treatment

讨论

All-on-4是对于终末期牙列成熟、有效的种植修复方式，往往可以避免植骨，且获得良好的初期稳定性并能够即刻负重，相对微创而又快速地为患者恢复咀嚼功能和美观效果。

All-on-4一般都需要较长种植体，尤其是斜行种植体长度至少需要14mm，对植入角度的把握有一定的难度。自由手种植往往需要大范围翻瓣，直视下清楚观察牙槽嵴方向，才能较准确地斜行植入较长的种植体。种植导板能够有效约束钻针及携带器的方向，可以在不翻瓣的情况下准确植入种植体，极大地为患者减少创伤。

Discussion

All-on-4 is a mature and effective implant restoration method for terminal dentition. It can often avoid bone grafting and obtain good primary stability and immediate loading. It is relatively minimally invasive and can quickly restore the masticatory function and aesthetic effect for patients.

Generally, the implants used in All-on-4 implants are quite long, especially the length of oblique implants needs to be at least 14mm, and it is difficult to control the insertion angle. Free-hand implants often require extensive flap and clear observation of the direction of the alveolar ridge under direct vision, in order to place long implants more accurately. The implant guided template can effectively restrain the direction of the drills and the implant carrier, so that the implant can be placed accurately without flap, which greatly reduces the trauma of the surgery.

病例5　无牙颌黏膜支持式先锋钻导板全口种植即刻修复一例

Case 5 Immediate Loading of Edentulous Jaws with Mucosa-supported Pioneer Drill-guided Templates: A Case Report

本病例资料由闫夏医生、刘海林技师提供，余涛医生整理

Provided from Dr. Xia Yan and Dt. Hailin Liu, and arranged by Dr. Tao Yu

初诊情况

基本信息：72岁男性。

主诉：上下颌全部牙齿缺失2个月。

现病史：2个月前，于外院拔除上下颌全部剩余牙齿，未曾修复，现无法咀嚼，咨询种植固定修复。

既往史：高血压，服药控制血压为130～140/80～90mmHg，否认冠心病。

检查：18-28、38-48缺失，剩余牙槽骨中度吸收，黏膜未见明显红肿。上下颌牙槽嵴覆盖关系基本正常，颌间距离不足（图2）。面下1/3无明显降低，上唇丰满度稍有不足，但仍属于可接受范围（图1）。

影像学检查：CBCT显示剩余牙槽骨骨量尚可。

诊断

上下颌牙列缺失。

Pretreatment

Basic information: 72-year-old man.

Chief complaint: All tooth loss in both upper and lower jaws for 2 months.

History of present illness: All the remaining teeth in the upper and lower jaws were extracted in another hospital 2 months ago, which had not been restored. Now, he could not chew and consulted for implant fixed restoration.

Past history: The patient's previous history of hypertension was controlled by medication (130-140/80-90mmHg), and coronary heart disease was denied.

Examination: He had a loss of 18-28, 38-48, moderate absorption of the remaining alveolar bone, and no obvious redness and swelling of the mucosa. The maxillary and mandibular alveolar ridge relationship was basically normal, and the intermaxillary distance was insufficient (Fig. 2). There was no significant reduction in the lower 1/3 of the face, and the fullness of the upper lip was slightly deficient but still within the acceptable range (Fig. 1).

Radiographic examination: CBCT showed that the amount of residual alveolar bone was acceptable (Figs. 8 to 15).

Diagnosis

Edentulous maxilla and mandible.

治疗计划

上下颌截骨，All-on-4种植，即刻过渡修复，3个月后永久修复。

术前准备

由于患者已缺失全部牙齿，目前缺乏咬合支持。因此先为患者制作了上下颌总义齿确定颌位关系，评估美学效果（图1），并注入X线阻射性材料，作为放射导板（图3），佩戴其再次进行CBCT扫描。将放射导板进行光学扫描，作为制作种植导板的数字模型，与CBCT一并导入导板设计软件。

分别于15、12、22、25位点设计植入Bredent SKY4.5mm×12mm、4.0mm×12mm、4.0mm×12mm、4.5mm×10mm种植体各一颗，分别于35、32、42、45位点植入Bredent SKY4.5mm×12mm、4.5mm×14mm、4.5mm×14mm、4.5mm×12mm种植体各一颗（图4、图5、图8～图15）。并于上下颌规划截骨线，放置两个固位钉指示截骨线位置。另外上下颌导板各自设计了3个固位钉。将设计完成的导板3D打印，粘接对应的导环，其中截骨位置使用红色导环特殊标记（图6）。

Treatment plan

Upper and lower jaw osteotomy, All-on-4 implant, immediate transitional restorations, and definitive restorations 3 months later.

Preoperative preparation

As the patient had lost all teeth, occlusal support was currently lacking. Therefore, the upper and lower complete dentures were made for the patient to determine the jaw relationship and evaluate the aesthetic effect (Fig. 1). The X-ray opaque material was injected to make radiation guides (Fig. 3), which were worn for CBCT scanning again. The optical scans of the radiation guides were used as digital models of the guided templates, which were imported into the guide design software together with CBCT.

For maxilla, Bredent SKY4.5×12mm, 4.0×12mm, 4.0×12mm and 4.5×10mm implants were designed at the 15, 12, 22, and 25 sites, respectively. For mandible, Bredent SKY 4.5×12mm, 4.5×14mm, 4.5×14mm, and 4.5×12mm implants were designed at the 35, 32, 42, and 45 sites, respectively (Figs. 4, 5, 8 to 15). Since osteotomy was required for both maxilla and mandible, two fixation pins were placed in each jaw to indicate the location of the osteotomy line. In addition, three fixation pins were designed and distributed in all anterior and posterior regions for each of the maxillary and mandibular guided templates. The designed guided template was 3D printed, and the corresponding guide rings were bonded. The osteotomy positions were marked with the red guide rings (Fig. 6).

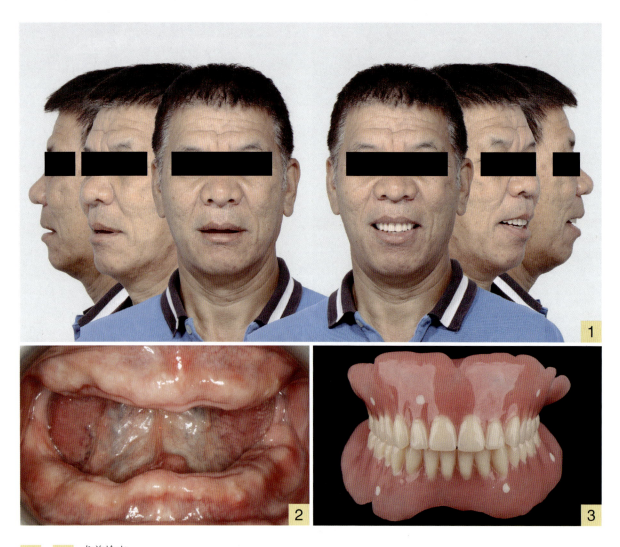

1 ~ 3 术前检查
Pretreatment examination

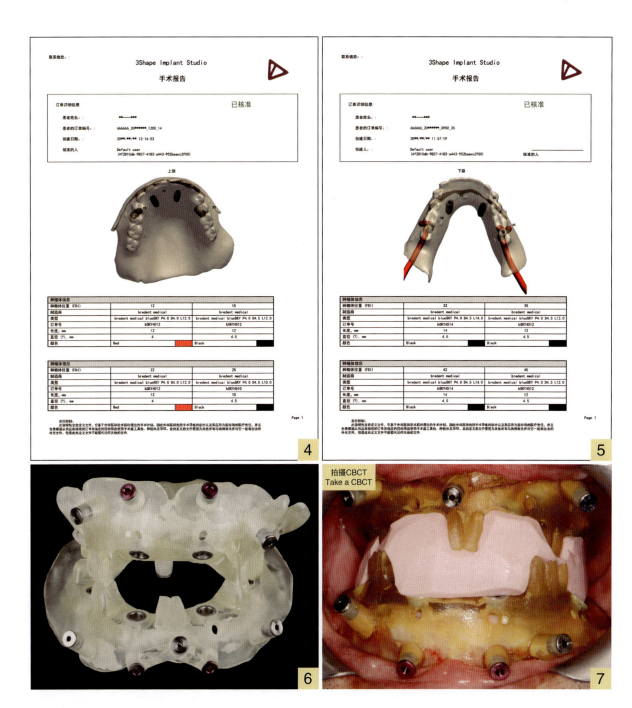

4 ~ 7 设计种植导板–1
The design of the surgical template-1

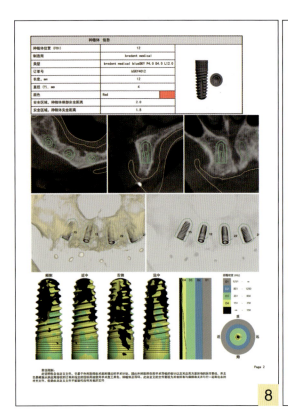

8

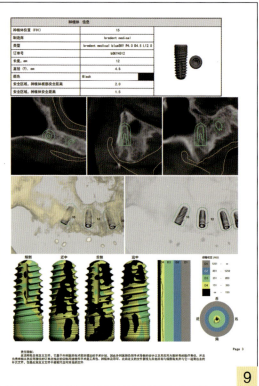

9

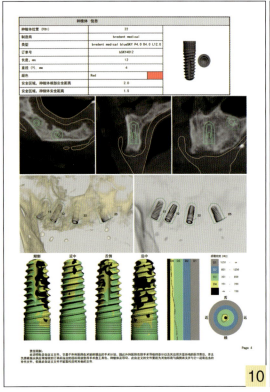

10

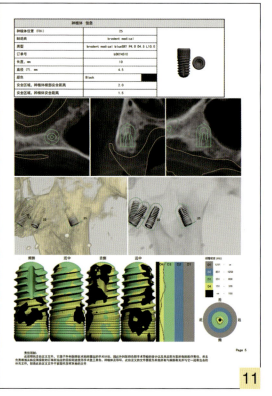

11

8 ~ 11 设计种植导板-2
The design of the surgical template-2

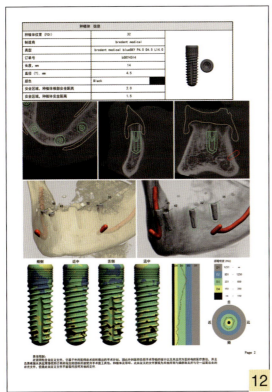

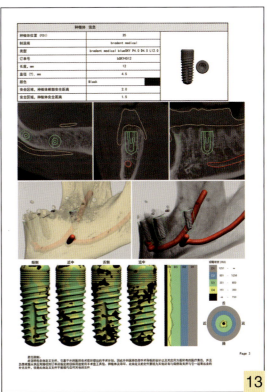

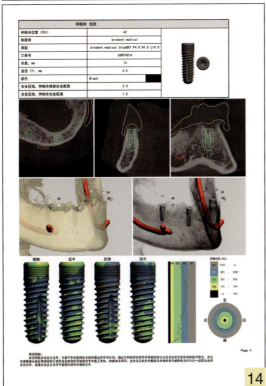

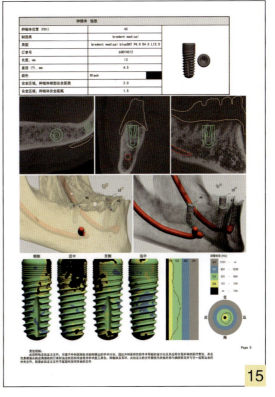

12 ~ 15 设计种植导板-3
The design of the surgical template-3

治疗过程

常规消毒铺巾后，上下颌牙槽嵴局部浸润麻醉，戴入上下颌种植导板，并使用硅橡胶咬合导板使之稳定（图7）。使用固位钉钻预备固位钉孔（图17），安装固位钉固定上下颌种植导板（图16和图33）。导板稳定后，在红色导环引导下预备截骨线指示孔，预备至止动环与导环完全接触，以确保指示孔贯穿牙槽嵴唇舌向全部厚度（图18）。使用对应长度的先锋钻，进行上下颌先锋钻预备（图19）。取下种植导板，沿牙槽嵴顶切开（图20和图34），翻瓣，充分暴露牙槽骨。将两个截骨线指示孔连成直线，则是设计的截骨线位置，使用超声骨刀截骨，并使用钨钢钻针修整牙槽骨锐利边缘（图21、图35和图36）。牙槽骨上先锋钻预备的窝洞清晰可见（图22），沿着这些窝洞，使用对应扩孔钻和止动环进行逐级备洞，并植入种植体，植入扭矩均达到45Ncm或者更高，初期稳定性良好（图23～图27、图37和图38）。安装Fast-Fix复合基台，上紧螺丝至25Ncm（图28、图29和图31）。安装复合基台保护帽，并用10Ncm的扭矩旋紧，骨缺损处植入骨粉恢复牙槽嵴轮廓（图30），再使用不可吸收线严密缝合，上下颌手术完成（图32、图39和图40）。

Treatment process

After routine disinfection, the maxillary and mandibular alveolar ridges were locally infiltrated under anesthesia, and the maxillary and mandibular implant guides were placed and stabilized with silicone rubber occlusal guides (Fig. 7). The fixation pin holes were prepared by using the fixation pin drilling (Fig. 17), and the fixation pins were installed to fix the maxillary and mandibular implant guide plates (Figs. 16 and 33). After the guide plate were seated, the osteotomy line indicator holes were prepared under the guidance of the red guide rings until the stop ring was completely in contact with the guide rings to ensure that the indicator holes penetrated the full thickness of the alveolar ridge in the labial and lingual directions (Fig. 18). Using the pioneer drill of the corresponding length, the upper and lower pioneer drill preparation was performed (Fig. 19). The implant guide plates were removed and an incisions were made along the crest of the alveolar ridge (Figs. 20 and 34), and the flaps was turned to fully expose the alveolar bone. The two osteotomy lines indicating the holes were connected into a straight line, which were the designed osteotomy line position. The osteotomy was performed with an ultrasonic osteotome, and the sharp edge of the alveolar bone was trimmed with a tungsten steel drill needle (Figs. 21, 35, and 36). The cavities prepared by the pioneer drill on the alveolar bone were clearly visible (Fig. 22). Along these cavities, the corresponding step drills and the stoppers were used to prepare the holes step by step, and the implants were implanted. The insertion torque reached 45Ncm or higher, and the initial stability was good (Figs. 23 to 27, 37, and 38). The fast-fix multi-unit abutments were tightened to 25Ncm (Figs. 28, 29, and 31), and covered by the protective caps with a torque of 10Ncm. Bone substitute was applied to regenerate the defected alveolar ridge (Fig. 30). Then the wounds were closed with non-absorbable sutures to complete the maxillary and mandibular surgeries (Figs. 32, 39, and 40).

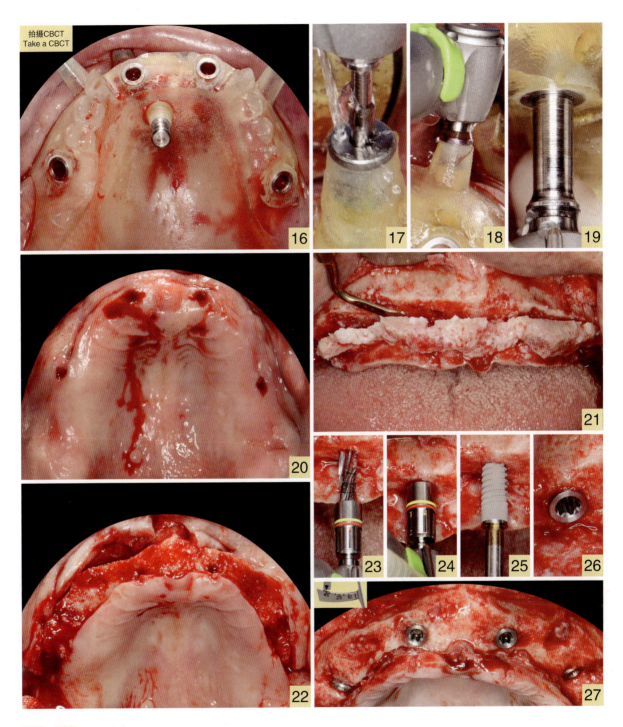

拍摄CBCT
Take a CBCT

16 ~ 27 上颌手术-1
The surgery of the maxilla-1

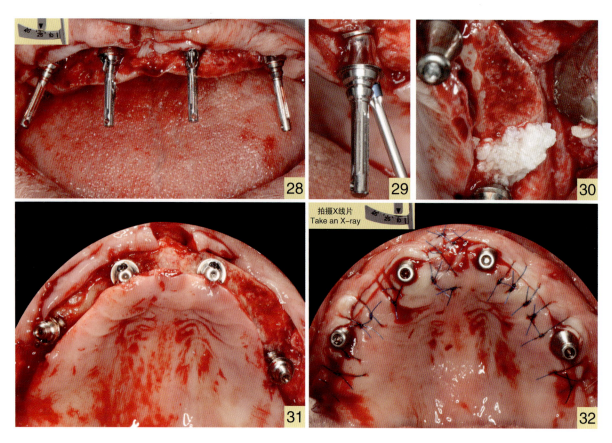

28 ~ 32　上颌手术–2
The surgery of the maxilla-2

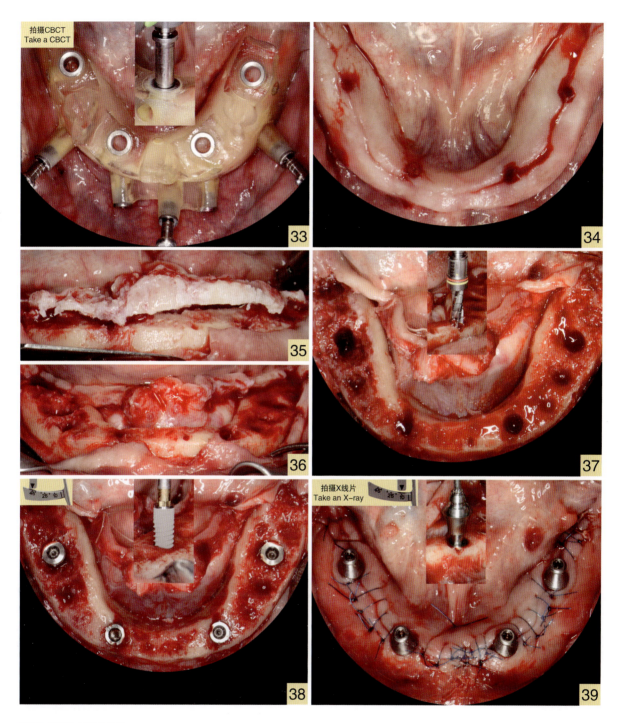

33 ~ 39 下颌手术
The surgery of the mandibular

拍片确认所有种植体位置良好，复合基台完全就位后，使用硅橡胶制取颌位记录，确定中线、𬌗平面（图41）。取下复合基台保护帽，安装复合基台水平转移杆，拍片确认转移杆完全就位，再使用牙科种植用连接件+成型树脂在口内连接（图42和图43），上下颌均使用硅橡胶制取开窗夹板式基台水平印模。再次安装复合基台保护帽。将印模转至技工室灌模型，上𬌗架，制作即刻过渡义齿。并于手术当天取下复合基台保护帽，为患者戴入即刻过渡义齿，拍片确认义齿完全就位（图44~图47）。

过渡修复3个月后，义齿稳定，种植体无松动，患者无不适主诉，对过渡修复效果较为满意（图48）。但是口腔卫生较差，尤其是下颌牙槽嵴改建，高度降低后，牙槽嵴与义齿组织面之间有明显的软垢堆积，牙槽嵴黏膜发红（图50和图52）。向患者加强口腔卫生宣教，教会牙缝刷使用，并在永久修复义齿外形设计时，考虑减小牙槽嵴与义齿之间的间隙，但也需要留出牙缝刷清洁通道。将所有复合基台再次加力至25Ncm，安装复合基台转移杆并用成型树脂于口内再次连接，使用个别托盘制取上下颌硅橡胶制取开窗夹板式基台水平印模，灌制石膏模型，用过渡义齿与硅橡胶制取咬合记录并将模型上𬌗架。为患者制作评估桥（图51），戴入口内后拍片确认完全就位（图53），评估桥中线、𬌗平面正确，前牙丰满度合适，垂直距离合适，正中关系正确，双侧咬合均匀稳定，患者对牙齿排列满意（图49）。

Radiographs were taken to confirm that all implants were in good position. After the multi-unit abutments was completely in place, silicone rubber was used to record the jaw position and determine the midline and occlusal plane (Fig. 41). The protective caps of the multi-unit abutments were removed, and the transfer copings of the multi-unit abutments were installed. The X-ray film was taken to confirm that the transfer copings were completely in place, then the steel pods and pattern resin were used to connect the transfer copings in the mouth (Figs. 42 and 43). The impressions of the abutments with splinted open-tray transfer copings were made with silicone on the upper and lower jaws. The multi-unit abutment protective caps were installed again. The impressions were sent to the lab to fill the models and mounted on an articulator to make the immediate transition restorations. On the day of surgery, the protective caps of the multi-unit abutments were removed, and the immediate transition restorations were delivered. X-ray Film was taken to confirm that the restorations were completely in place (Figs. 44 to 47).

After 3 months of transitional restoration, the restorations were stable, no loosening of the implant was found, and the patient had no complaints of discomfort and was satisfied with the effect of transitional restoration (Fig. 48). However, the oral hygiene was long, especially for the reconstruction of the mandibular alveolar ridge. After the height was reduced, there was obvious soft scale accumulation between the alveolar ridge and the tissue surface of the restoration, and the mucosa of the alveolar ridge became red (Figs. 50 and 52). Oral hygiene instruction should be emphasized to the patients, and the use of interdental brush should be taught. In the shape design of the definitive restorations, it was considered to reduce the gap between the alveolar ridge and the restoration, but it was also necessary to leave a clean channel for the interdental brush. All the abutments were re-forced to 25Ncm, and the multi-unit abutments transfer copings were installed and re-connected with pattern resin in the mouth. The impressions of the upper and lower jaw were made with silicone rubber, and the plaster casts were filled. An evaluation bridges were made for the patient (Fig. 51), and the X-ray was taken to confirm that them

用硅橡胶翻制评估桥外形印模（图54）。光学扫描评估桥并数字化复制其外形，并回切全瓷牙冠及牙龈部分烤塑空间（图55和图56）。切削PMMA支架，验证回切空间合适（图57、图58和图61）。切削正式钛架，并确认全瓷牙冠修复及牙龈部分烤塑空间合适（图59、图60和图62）。钛架表面遮色，光学扫描，设计16-26、36-46全瓷冠，并用高透渐变色氧化锆制作全锆冠，前磨牙及磨牙仅进行外染色而不加饰瓷，前牙进行少量回切加饰瓷和上釉（图69、图63~图68）。牙龈部分进行烤塑，模拟天然牙龈颜色（图70~图72）。义齿组织面高度抛光，并留出牙缝刷清洁通道（图73和图74）。义齿再上殆架进行调殆，抛光（图75~图80）。完成的义齿前牙切端具有类似天然牙的半透明性，义齿整体质地、颜色自然（图81和图82）。

were completely in place (Fig. 53). It was evaluated that the middle line and occlusal plane of the bridge were correct, the fullness of the anterior teeth was appropriate, the vertical distance was appropriate, the median relationship was correct, the bilateral occlusion was uniform and stable, and the patient was satisfied with the arrangement of the teeth (Fig. 49).

Silicone rubber indexes were made for the evaluation bridges (Fig. 54). The evaluation bridges were optical scanned, and their shapes were digitally reduced to make space for ceramic crowns and the gingival molding (Figs. 55 and 56). The PMMA frameworks were milled to verify that the back cut spaces were suitable (Figs. 57, 58, and 61). The definitive titanium frameworks were milled. It was confirmed with the silicone indexes that the spaces for crowns and gingiva were adequate (Figs. 59, 60, and 62). The surfaces of the titanium frameworks were masked and optical scanned, and the 16-26 and 36-46 all ceramic crowns were designed. The all-zirconia crowns were fabricated with high transparence and gradient color zirconia. The premolars and molars were only externally stained without porcelain, and the anterior teeth were slightly cut back with porcelain and glazing (Figs. 69, 63 to 68). The gingival parts were baked with plastic to simulate the natural gingival color (Figs. 70 to 72). The tissue surfaces of the restorations were highly polished, and the interdental brushes were allowed to go through the cleaning channels (Figs. 73 and 74). The restorations were then put on the articulator for occlusal adjustment (Figs. 75 to 80). The incisor end of the finished restorations had a translucency similar to that of natural teeth, and the overall texture and color of the restorations were natural (Figs. 81 and 82).

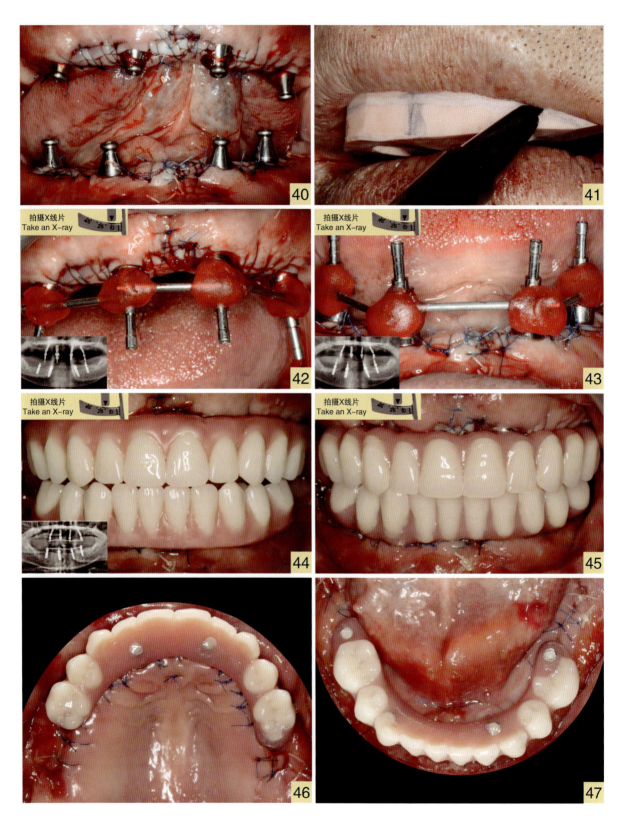

拍摄X线片
Take an X-ray

40 ~ 47 过渡修复体制作与戴牙
Fabrication and delivery of the immediate restorations

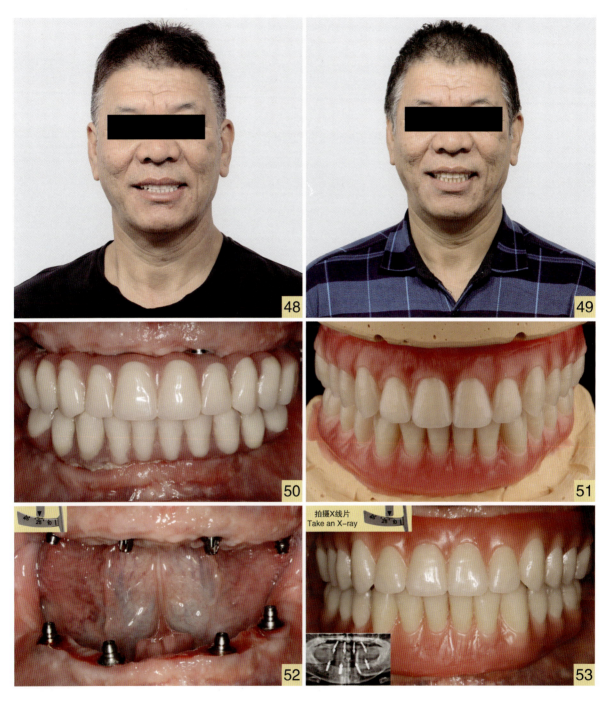

48 ~ 53 试戴评估桥
Try-in of evaluation bridge

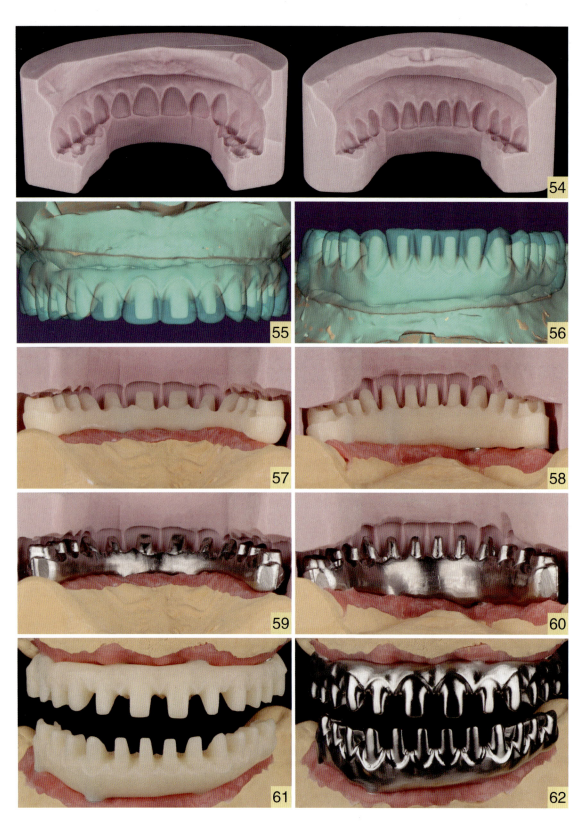

54 ~ 62　制作钛桥架
Machined titanium frameworks

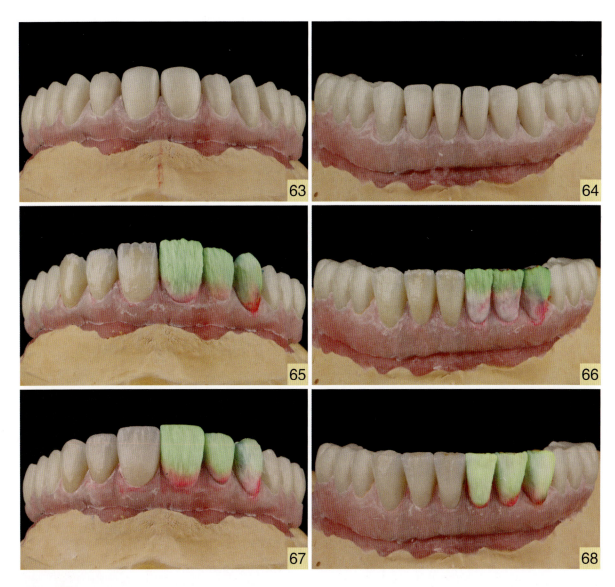

63 ~ 68 外冠烤瓷
Porcelain fused on the crowns

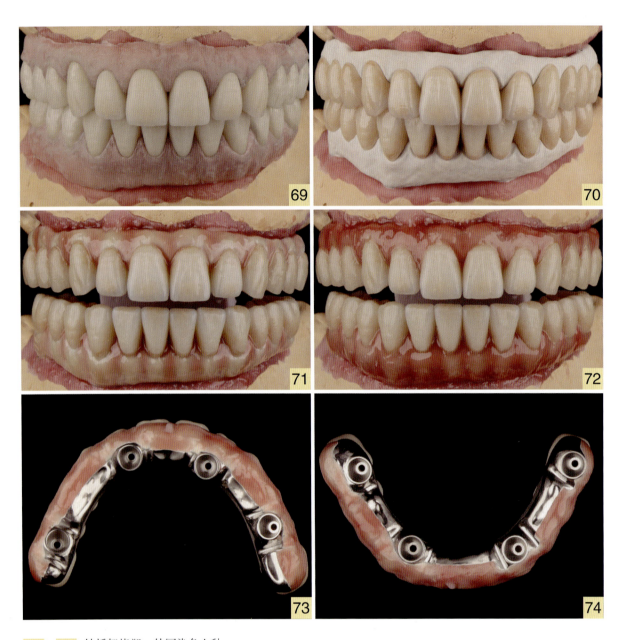

69 ~ 74 钛桥架烤塑，外冠染色上釉
Veneered titanium framework, staining and glazing on crowns

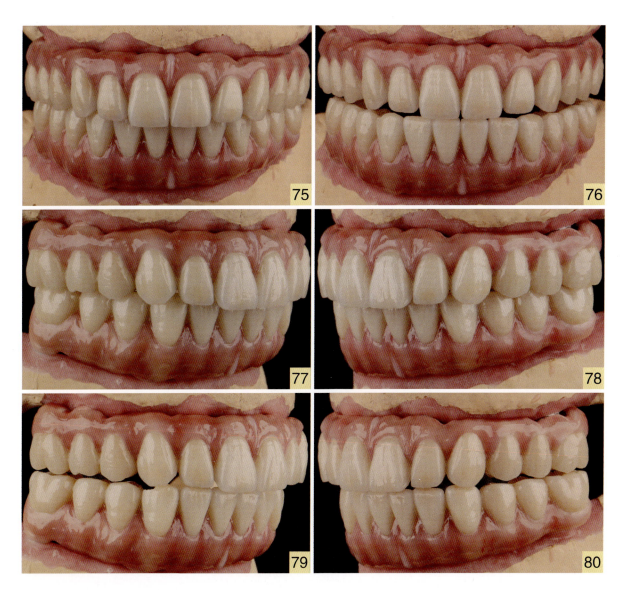

75 ～ 80 粭架上的完成义齿
Finished restorations on articulator

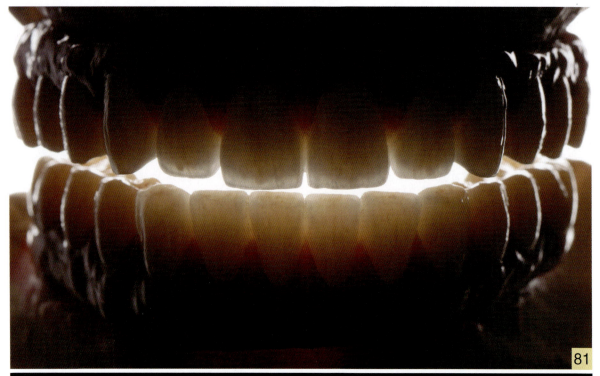

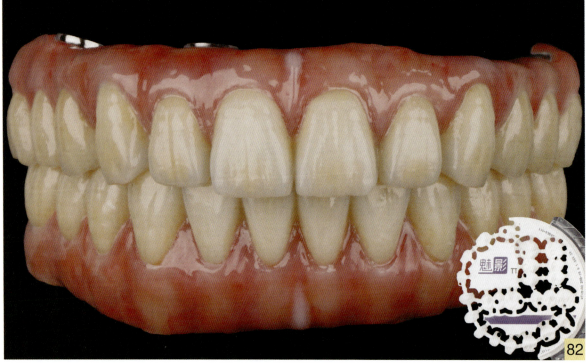

81，82 具有良好半透明性和色泽的完成义齿
Finished restorations with good translucence and color

在强化口腔卫生宣教后，患者通过自身努力，口腔卫生有较大改善，牙槽黏膜已没有明显红肿（图84）。将义齿于患者口内试戴，上紧二级螺丝至18Ncm，并拍摄X线片确定义齿完全就位（图85）。使用聚四氟乙烯膜+流动树脂封闭螺丝孔（图86和图87）。在患者口内调𬌗，正中𬌗双侧后牙均匀接触，前伸𬌗多个前牙均匀接触而后牙脱离接触，侧方𬌗工作侧为组牙功能𬌗（图88～图93）。再次抛光义齿，完成修复（图94和图95）。患者获得了良好的咀嚼功能和美观效果（图83和图97），义齿组织面保留了良好的清洁通道（图96）。

讨论

无牙颌患者设计种植导板需要先制作放射导板，制取正确的颌位关系，确认牙齿排列的美学效果。只有在这种情况下，才能准确评估修复间隙是否充足，才能准确判断是否需要截骨以及截骨量的大小。参照放射导板提供的正确修复体信息，才能进行正确的种植设计。

截骨操作需要翻瓣进行，也意味着这是一台翻瓣手术，术者可以直视下看到牙槽骨的形态。先锋钻导板确定种植位点，提供初步的种植角度和深度参考，可大大降低自由手完成后续的备洞和种植体植入的难度。最终种植体植入的位置和角度正确，获得良好的种植修复效果。

After emphasizing the oral hygiene education, the patient's oral hygiene was greatly improved through his own efforts, and the alveolar mucosa had no obvious redness and swelling (Fig. 84). The restorations were tried in the patient's mouth, the secondary screw was tightened to 18Ncm, and the X-ray film was taken to confirm that the restorations were completely in place (Fig. 85). The screw holes were closed using PTFE membrane + flowable resin (Figs. 86 and 87). In the patient's mouth, the posterior teeth on both sides were in uniform contact in centric occlusion. The multiple anterior teeth were in uniform guidance with the posterior teeth and out of contact in protrusive occlusion. The lateral occlusions of both sides were group functional occlusion (Figs. 88 to 93). The restorations were polished again to be finalized (Figs. 94 and 95). The patient obtained good masticatory function and aesthetic results (Figs. 83 and 97), and the tissue surface of the restorations remained good cleaning accesses (Fig. 96).

Discussion

Surgical templates for edentulous patients require the fabrication of radiation guides for implant placement, obtaining the correct jaw relationship, and confirming the aesthetic outcome of tooth arrangement. Only under these circumstances, can the adequacy of the restorative space be accurately evaluated, and the need for bone resection and the amount of bone resected can be accurately determined. Referring to the correct restorative information provided by the radiation guides, accurate implant planning can be achieved.

The osteotomy procedure needs to be flap-turnover, which means it is a flap surgery, allowing the surgeon to directly visualize the morphology of the alveolar bone. The use of a pilot drill guide determines the implant site, providing initial reference for implant angle and depth, which can greatly reduce the difficulty of subsequent drilling and implant placement by freehand. Ultimately, correct implant positioning and angle result in a good implant restoration effect.

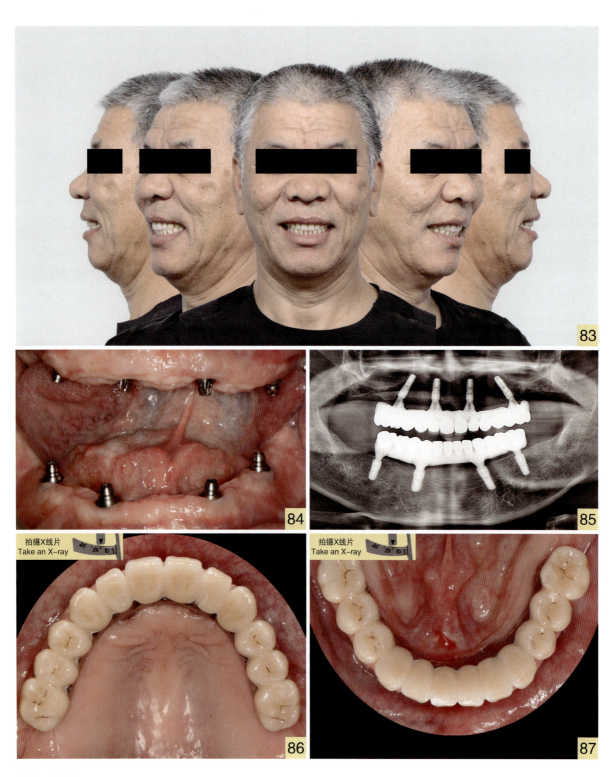

83 ~ 87 戴永久义齿-1
Delivery of the definitive restorations-1

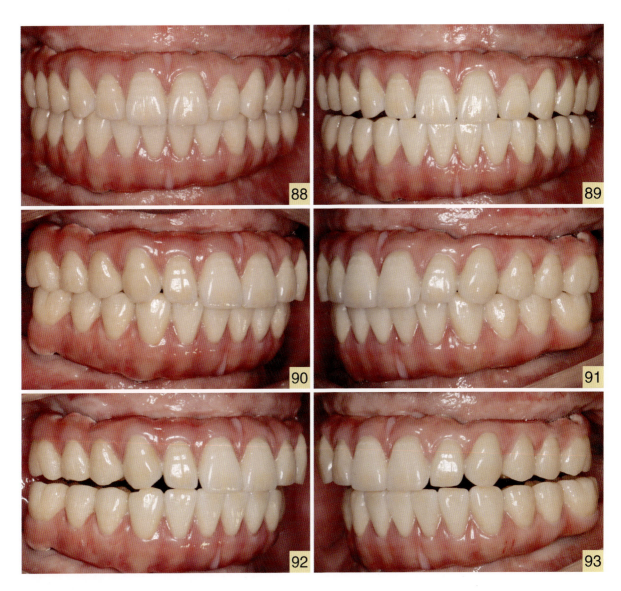

88 ~ 93 戴永久义齿-2
Delivery of the definitive restorations-2

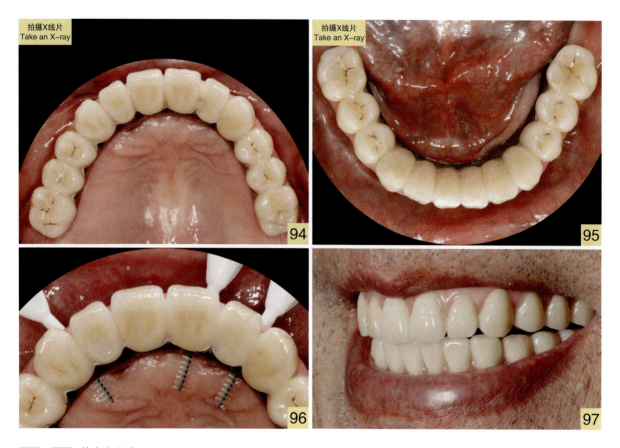

94 ~ 97 戴永久义齿-3
Delivery of the definitive restorations-3

病例6　无牙颌黏膜支持式上颌半程导板、下颌全程导板全口种植即刻修复一例

Case 6 Immediate Implant-supported Full-mouth Rehabilitation with Half-guided Template for Maxilla and Full-guided Template for Mandible: A Case Report

本病例资料由丁明会医生、刘海林技师提供，余涛医生整理

Provided from Dr. Minghui Ding and Dt. Hailin Liu, and arranged by Dr. Tao Yu

初诊情况

基本信息：61岁女性。

主诉：上下颌多数牙缺失10余年。

现病史：10余年以来，上下颌多颗牙缺失，曾于外院活动义齿修复，戴用不便，且近期又有牙齿缺失，旧义齿不能戴用，无法咀嚼，咨询种植固定修复。

既往史：无特殊。

检查：18-28、38-47缺失，剩余牙槽骨中度吸收，黏膜未见明显红肿。48近中倾斜，龋坏，叩痛（－），松动Ⅰ度，牙龈无红肿。上下颌牙槽嵴覆盖关系基本正常，颌间距离基本正常（图1～图4）。

影像学检查：曲面体层片显示48牙槽骨吸收至根中1/3，根尖周未见明显透射影；上颌前磨牙区、前牙区牙槽骨高度尚可，双侧上颌窦气化明显，双侧上颌磨牙区牙槽骨高度不足；下颌剩余牙槽骨高度尚可（图5）。

Pretreatment

Basic information: 61-year-old female.

Chief complaint: Most of the upper and lower teeth were missing for more than 10 years.

History of present illness: For more than 10 years, a number of teeth in the upper and lower jaws were missing, and had been restored with removable dentures in another hospital, which was inconvenient to wear. Moreover, the old dentures could not be worn and could not chew due to tooth loss recently.

Past history: No special history.

Examination: It revealed teeth missing from 18 to 28 and 38 to 47, moderate absorption of the remaining alveolar bone, and no obvious redness or swelling of the mucosa. 48 was mesial tilted and decayed with no percussion pain, redness or swelling of the gingiva. The maxillary and mandibular alveolar ridge relationship was almost normal, and the intermaxillary distance was almost normal (Figs. 1 to 4).

Radiographic examination: It showed that the alveolar bone was absorbed into the middle 1/3 of the root in 48, and no obvious radiations were observed around the apex. The alveolar bone height of the maxillary premolar and anterior teeth was acceptable, but the bilateral maxillary sinus pneumatization was obvious. The alveolar bone height of the bilateral maxillary molars was insufficient. The height of the residual alveolar bone in the mandible was acceptable (Fig. 5).

诊断

上颌牙列缺失，下颌牙列缺损，48牙体缺损。

治疗计划

拔除48，上下颌All-on-6种植，即刻过渡修复，3个月后永久修复。

术前准备

由于患者已丧失几乎全部牙齿，目前缺乏咬合支持。因此先为患者制作了上下颌总义齿确定颌位关系，评估美学效果（图6和图7），并注入X线阻射性材料，作为放射导板，佩戴其再次进行CBCT扫描。将放射导板进行光学扫描，作为制作种植导板的数字模型，与CBCT一并导入导板设计软件。

按照表1于上下颌各个位点设计植入种植体（图9和图10）。

表1 计划植入的种植体

牙位	种植体品牌	尺寸
16	Bredent SKY	4.5mm × 14mm
14	Bredent SKY	4.0mm × 14mm
12	Bredent SKY	3.5mm × 12mm
22	Bredent SKY	3.5mm × 12mm
24	Bredent SKY	4.0mm × 12mm
26	Bredent SKY	4.5mm × 12mm
36	Bredent SKY	4.5mm × 10mm
34	Bredent SKY	4.0mm × 12mm
32	Bredent SKY	3.5mm × 12mm
42	Bredent SKY	3.5mm × 12mm
44	Bredent SKY	4.0mm × 12mm
46	Bredent SKY	4.5mm × 10mm

Diagnosis

Complete edentulous maxilla, partial edentulous mandible, 48 tooth defect.

Treatment plan

48 extracted, upper and lower jaw All-on-6 implants, immediate transitional restorations, and definitive restorations 3 months later.

Preoperative preparation

Occlusal support was currently lacking because the patient had lost almost all her teeth. Therefore, the upper and lower complete dentures were made for the patient to determine the jaw relationship and evaluate the aesthetic effect (Figs. 6 and 7), and the X-ray radiation shielding material was injected to make a radiation guide plate, which was worn for CBCT scanning again. Optical scanning of the radiation guides was performed as digital models of the implant guided templates, which were imported into the guide design software together with CBCT.

According to Table 1, the implants were designed and placed at each site of the upper and lower jaw (Figs. 9 and 10).

Table 1　Planned implants

Position of teeth	Brand of implant	Size
16	Bredent SKY	4.5×14mm
14	Bredent SKY	4.0×14mm
12	Bredent SKY	3.5×12mm
22	Bredent SKY	3.5×12mm
24	Bredent SKY	4.0×12mm
26	Bredent SKY	4.5×12mm
36	Bredent SKY	4.5×10mm
34	Bredent SKY	4.0×12mm
32	Bredent SKY	3.5×12mm
42	Bredent SKY	3.5×12mm
44	Bredent SKY	4.0×12mm
46	Bredent SKY	4.5×10mm

由于上颌磨牙区牙槽骨高度不足，16种植体颈部斜向远中，根尖部避开右侧上颌窦，26种植体根尖部斜向远中避开左侧上颌窦。其余种植位点牙槽骨骨量及角度尚可，均设计为直立植入种植体（图15～图26）。并于上下颌各设计4个固位钉，增加种植导板稳定性和固位力。将设计完成的导板3D打印，粘接对应的导环（图8、图11和图12），准备导板手术工具盒（图13）。

治疗过程

常规消毒铺巾后，上下颌牙槽嵴局部浸润麻醉，微创拔除48，戴入上下颌种植导板，并使用硅橡胶咬合导板使之稳定，使用固位钉钻预备固位钉孔（图14），安装固位钉固定上颌种植导板（图27）。在种植导板引导下逐级备洞。完成窝洞预备后，取下上颌种植导板，沿牙槽嵴顶切开、翻瓣，按照计划沿着制备的窝洞植入各个位点对应的种植体，植入扭矩均达到45Ncm或者更高，初期稳定性良好（图28和图29、图33～图38）。然后安装Fast-Fix复合基台，上紧螺丝至25Ncm（图30）。安装复合基台保护帽，并用10Ncm的扭矩旋紧（图31），修整并复位软组织瓣，严密缝合（图32），上颌手术完成。

Due to insufficient alveolar bone height in the maxillary molar region, the implant of 16 was tilted distally and the apical part avoided the right maxillary sinus, while the apical part of 26 implants was tilted distally to avoid the left maxillary sinus. The rest of the implant sites had acceptable alveolar bone mass and angle, and were designed to place the implants in an upright position (Figs. 15 to 26). Four fixation pins were designed in the upper and lower jaws to increase the stability and retention force of the implant guided templates. The designed guided templates were 3D printed, the corresponding guide rings were bonded (Figs. 8, 11, and 12), and the surgical tool box of the guide plate was prepared (Fig. 13).

Treatment process

After routine disinfection and drape, the maxillary and mandibular alveolar ridge was locally infiltrated with anesthesia, and minimally invasive extraction 48 was performed. The maxillary and mandibular implant guided templates were placed and stabilized with silicone rubber occlusal guidance. The fixation pin holes were prepared with drills (Fig. 14). The maxillary implant guide plates were fixed with fixation pins (Fig. 27). After the cavity preparation was completed, the maxillary implant guide plate was removed, the alveolar crest was incised, flap was turned, and the corresponding implants were placed along the prepared cavities according to the plan. The insertion torque reached 45Ncm or higher, and the initial stability was good (Figs. 28, 29, 33 to 38). The fast-fix multi- unit abutments were then installed, and the screws were tightened to 25Ncm (Fig. 30). The multi-unit abutments protective caps were installed and tightened with a torque of 10Ncm (Fig. 31), the soft tissue flap was trimmed and reset, tightly sutured (Fig. 32), and the maxillary surgery was completed.

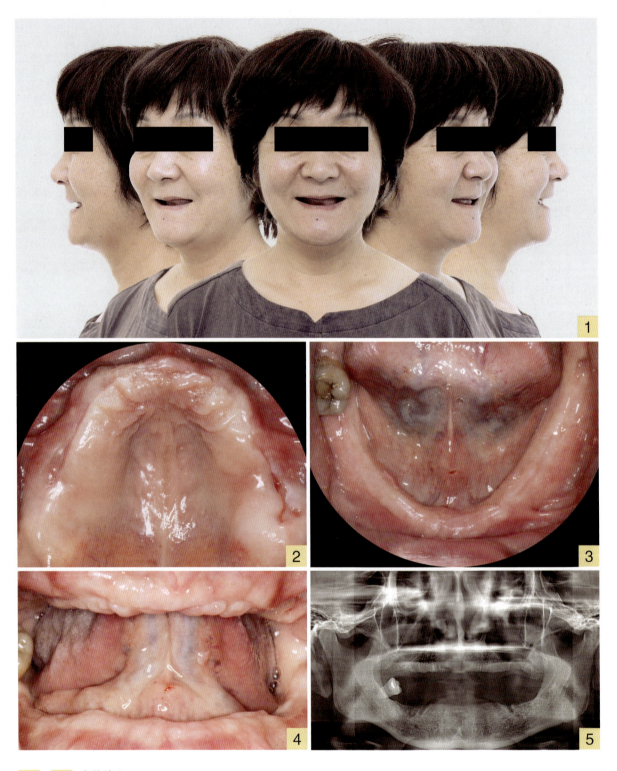

1 ~ 5 术前检查-1
Pretreatment examination-1

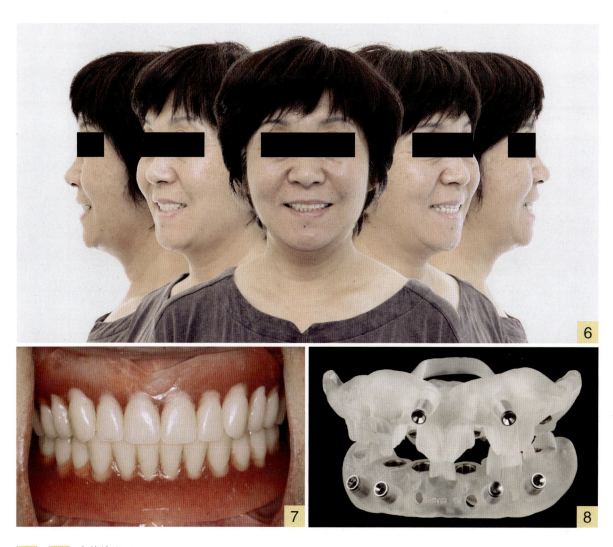

6 ~ 8 术前检查–2
Pretreatment examination-2

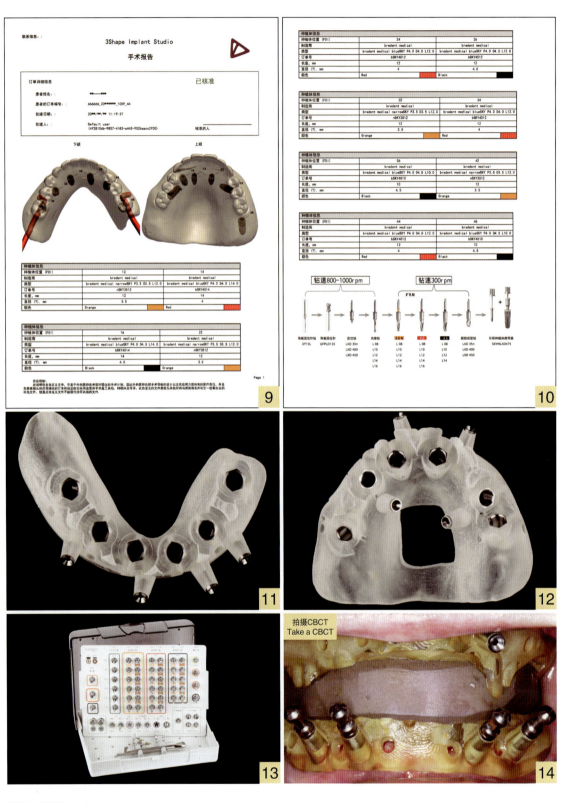

9 ~ 14 设计种植导板–1
The design of the surgical template-1

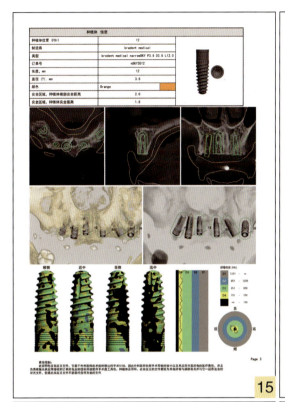

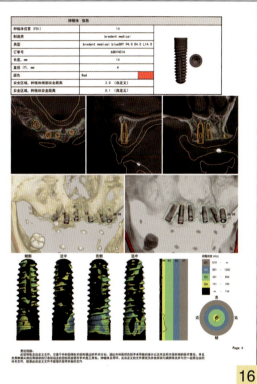

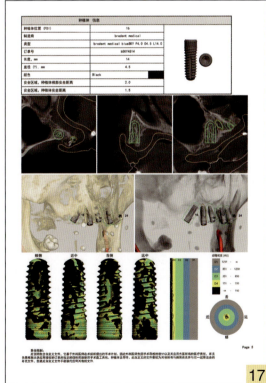

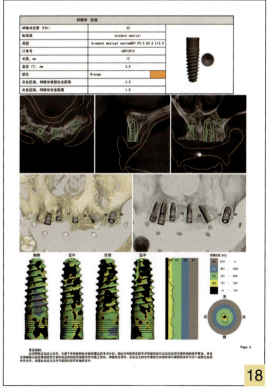

15~18 设计种植导板-2
The design of the surgical template-2

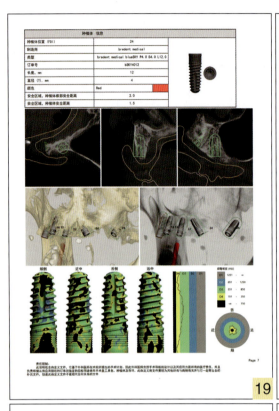
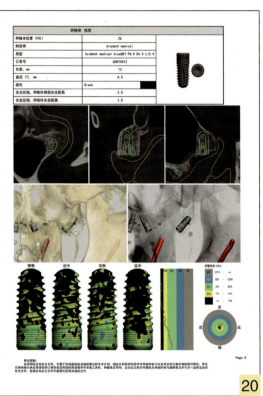
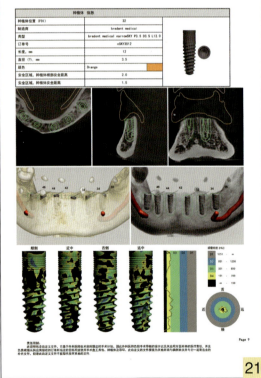
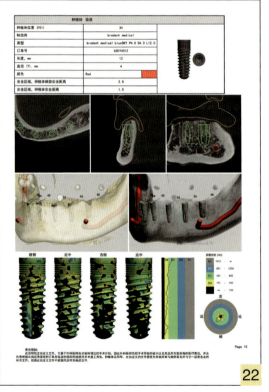

19~22　设计种植导板-3
The design of the surgical template-3

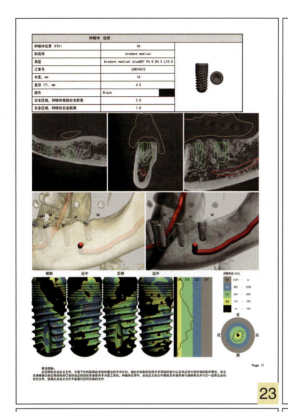

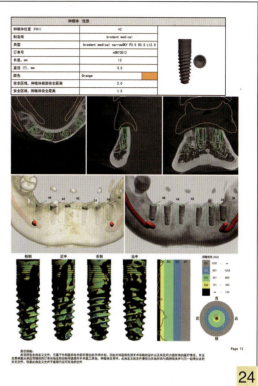

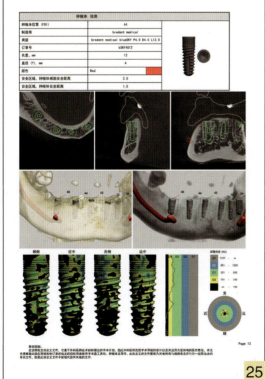

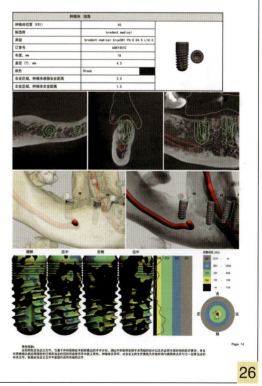

23 ~ 26 设计种植导板-4
The design of the surgical template-4

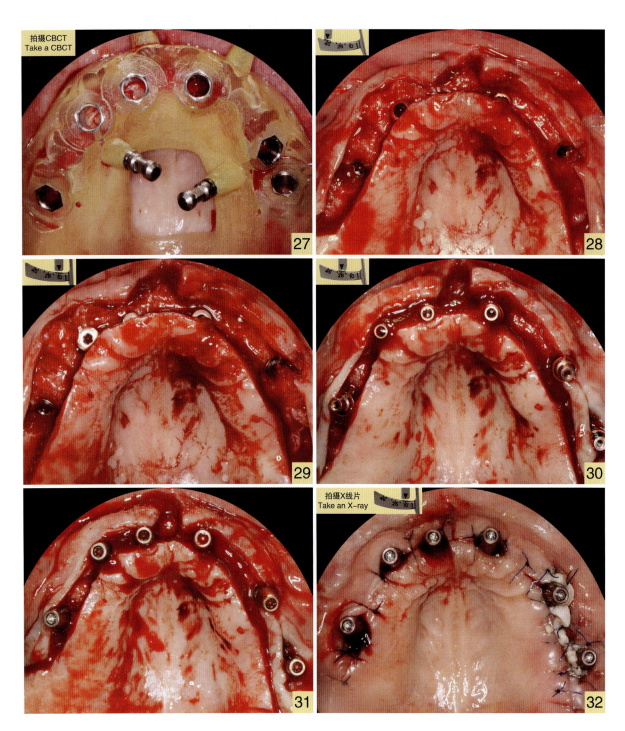

27 ~ 32　上颌术中概览
Overview of the surgery of the maxilla

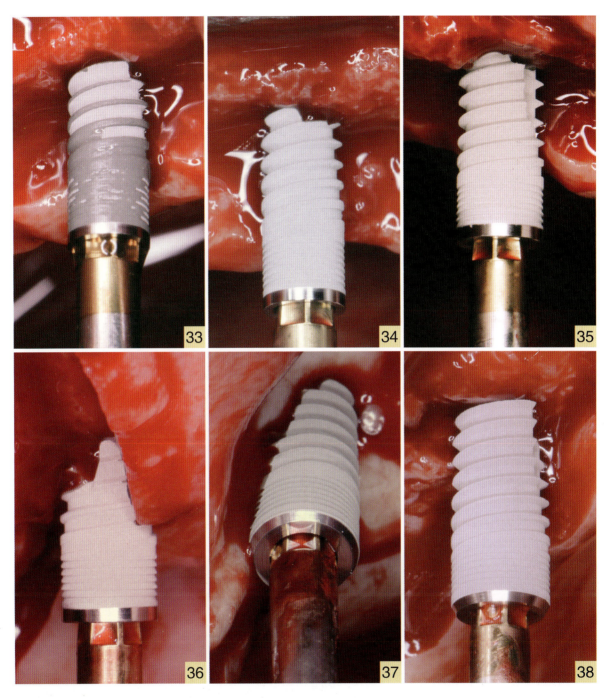

33 ~ 38 上颌术中细节
Details of the surgery of the maxilla

为了尽量保护下颌牙槽嵴角化黏膜，下颌种植窝洞预备之前，先沿牙槽嵴顶切开，小范围翻瓣，暴露牙槽嵴顶，减少窝洞预备时钻针对黏膜的损伤（图40）。再次通过固位钉将下颌种植导板固定（图39）。在种植导板引导下逐级备洞（图45和图46），并在种植导板引导下植入种植体（图47~图52、图41和图42）。然后安装Fast-Fix复合基台，上紧螺丝至25Ncm（图43）。安装复合基台保护帽，并用10Ncm的扭矩旋紧（图44），修整并复位软组织瓣，严密缝合，每个复合基台周围都有宽度不低于2mm的角化黏膜（图44），下颌手术完成。

拍片确认所有种植体位置良好，复合基台完全就位后，使用硅橡胶制取颌位记录，确定中线、𬌗平面。取下复合基台保护帽，安装复合基台水平转移杆，拍片确认转移杆完全就位，再使用牙科种植用连接件+成型树脂在口内连接，上下颌均使用硅橡胶制取开窗夹板式基台水平印模。再次安装复合基台保护帽。将印模转至技工室灌模型，上𬌗架，制作即刻过渡义齿。并于手术当天取下复合基台保护帽，为患者戴入即刻过渡义齿，二级螺丝旋紧至18Ncm（图54~图56），拍片确认义齿完全就位（图57），即刻为患者恢复咀嚼功能，改善牙齿美观（图53）。

In order to protect the keratinized mucosa of the mandibular alveolar ridge as much as possible, before the mandibular implant cavity preparation, the alveolar crest was incised along the alveolar crest, and a small area of flap was performed to expose the alveolar crest, so as to reduce the damage of the mucosa during the cavity preparation (Fig. 40). The mandibular implant guided template was again placed through the fixation pins (Fig. 39). The holes were prepared step by step under the guidance of the template (Figs. 45 and 46), and the implants were placed under the guidance of the template (Figs. 47 to 52, 41, 42). Then the fast-fix multi-unit abutments were installed, and the screws were tightened to 25Ncm (Fig. 43). The protective caps of the multi-unit abutments were installed with a torque of 10Ncm (Fig. 44). The soft tissue flap was trimmed and sutured to finish the mandibular surgery. The surrounding keratinized mucosa of each multi-unit abutment was no less than 2mm in width (Fig. 44).

Radiographs were taken to confirm that all implants were in good position and the multi-unit abutments were completely in place. Then silicone rubber was used to record jaw position, and the midline and occlusal plane were determined. The protective caps of the multi-unit abutments were removed, and the transfer copings of the multi-unit abutments were installed with a confirmation of seating by the X-ray film. The steel pods and pattern resin were used to connect the transfer copings in the mouth to take a splinted silicone impression. The multi-unit abutment protective caps were installed again. The technician fabricated the interim restorations in a rapid method. On the day of surgery, the protective caps of the multi-unit abutments were removed, and the immediate interim restorations were placed in the patient's mouth. The secondary screws were tightened to 18Ncm (Figs. 54 to 56), and the restorations were confirmed to be completely in place (Fig. 57) to regain the masticatory function and improve esthetics immediately (Fig. 53) .

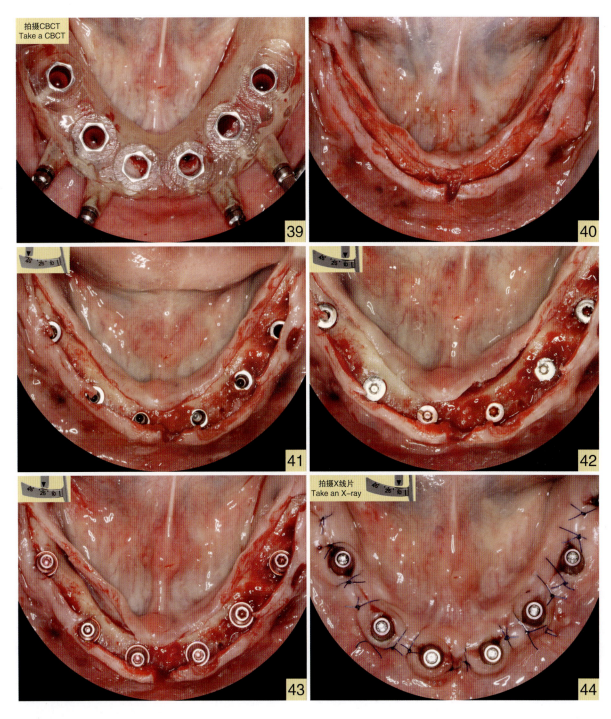

拍摄CBCT
Take a CBCT

39

40

41

42

拍摄X线片
Take an X-ray

43

44

39 ~ 44 下颌术中概览
Overview of the surgery of the mandibular

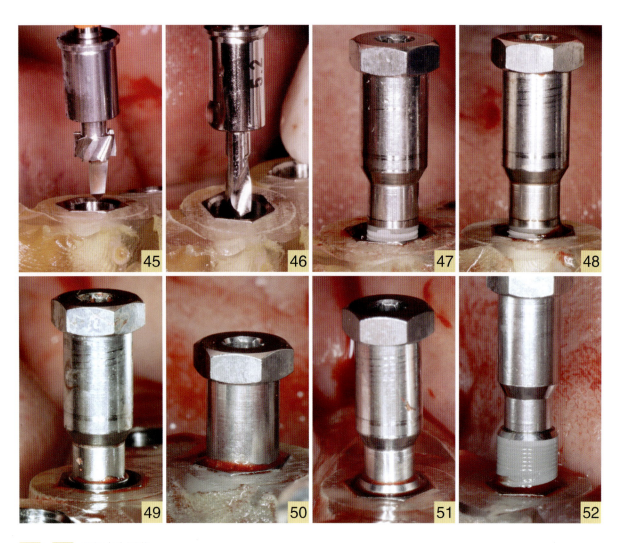

45 ~ 52 下颌术中细节
Details of the surgery of the mandibular

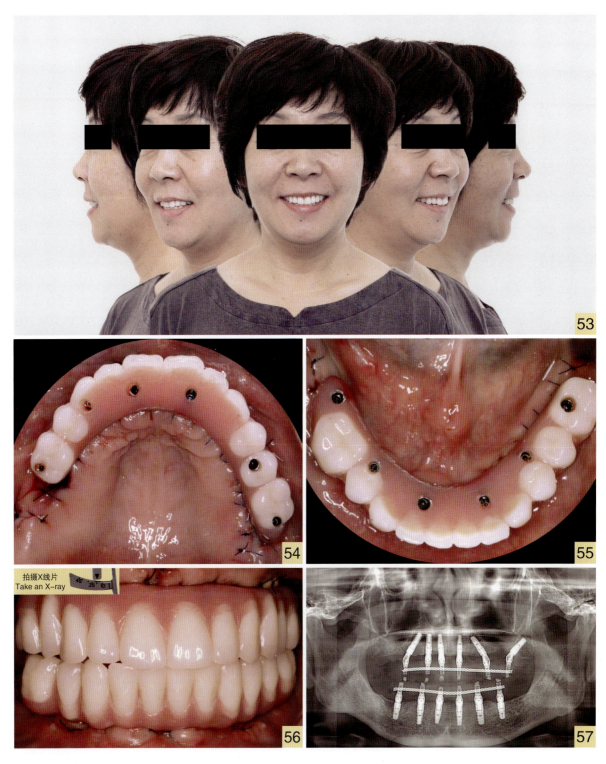

53 ~ 57 戴过渡修复体
Delivery of the immediate restorations

过渡修复3个月后，患者无不适主诉，对过渡修复效果较为满意（图58），检查发现过渡义齿稳定，种植体无松动（图60），拍摄曲面体层片显示种植体周围牙槽骨稳定，未见明显低密度影（图62）。取下过渡义齿，将所有复合基台再次加力至25Ncm，安装复合基台转移杆并用成型树脂于口内再次连接，使用个别托盘制取上下颌硅橡胶制取开窗夹板式基台水平印模，灌制石膏模型，用过渡义齿与硅橡胶制取咬合记录并将模型上𬌗架。为患者制作评估桥，戴入口内后拍片确认完全就位（图63），评估桥中线、𬌗平面正确，前牙丰满度合适，垂直距离合适，正中关系正确，双侧咬合均匀稳定，患者对牙齿排列满意（图59和图61）。

用硅橡胶翻制评估桥外形印模（图64）。光学扫描评估桥并数字化复制其外形，并回切全瓷牙冠及牙龈部分烤塑空间（图65和图66）。切削PMMA支架，验证回切空间合适（图67、图68和图71）。切削正式钛架，并确认全瓷牙冠修复及牙龈部分烤塑空间合适（图69、图70和图72）。钛架表面遮色，光学扫描，设计16-26、36-46全瓷冠，并用高透渐变色氧化锆制作全锆冠，仅进行外染色而不加饰瓷（图73和图74）。牙龈部分进行烤塑，模拟天然牙龈颜色（图75和图76）。义齿表面高度抛光，并在组织面留出牙缝刷清洁通道（图77～图80）。义齿再上𬌗架进行调𬌗，抛光（图81～图86）。

After 3 months, the patient had no complaints of discomfort and was satisfied with the effect of the transitional restorations (Fig. 58). The examination showed that the transitional restorations were stable and the implants were not loose (Fig. 60). Panoramic tomography showed that the alveolar bone around the implants was stable and no obvious low-density shadow was found (Fig. 62). After the transition restorations were removed, all the multi-unit abutments were re-forced to 25Ncm, and the multi-unit abutments transfer bars were installed and re-connected with pattern resin in the mouth. The impressions of the upper and lower jaw were made with silicone rubber using individual trays, and the plaster casts were filled. Evaluation bridges were made for the patient, and radiographs were taken to confirm that the bridges were completely in place (Fig. 63). It was evaluated that the middle line and occlusal plane of the bridges was correct, the fullness of the anterior teeth was appropriate, the vertical dimension was appropriate, the centric relationship was correct, the bilateral occlusion was uniform and stable, and the patient was satisfied with the tooth arrangement (Figs. 59 and 61).

The silicone rubber indexes recorded the shapes of the evaluation bridges (Fig. 64). The evaluation bridges were optical scanned. Cut back was made to provide the spaces for all ceramic crowns and part of the gingiva (Figs. 65 and 66). The PMMA frameworks were milled to verify that the back cut space was suitable (Figs. 67, 68, and 71). The formal titanium frameworks were machined, and it was confirmed that the full ceramic crowns and the gingival part plastic space were appropriate (Figs. 69, 70, and 72). The surfaces of the titanium frameworks were opaque, and optical scanning was used to design 16-26 and 36-46 all ceramic crowns. The all-zirconia crowns were made with high transparence gradient zirconia, and only external staining was performed without porcelain decoration (Figs. 73 and 74). The gingival part was veneered with plastic to simulate the natural gingival color (Figs. 75 and 76). The surfaces of the restorations were highly polished, and interdental brush cleaning channels were left on the tissue surface (Figs. 77 to 80). The restorations were then put on the articulator for occlusal adjustment and final polishing (Figs. 81 to 86).

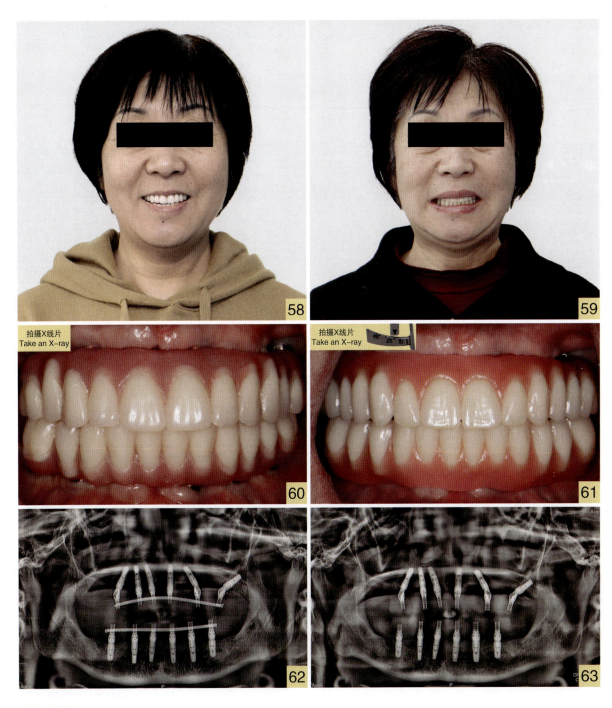

58 ~ 63　试戴评估桥
Try-in of evaluation bridge

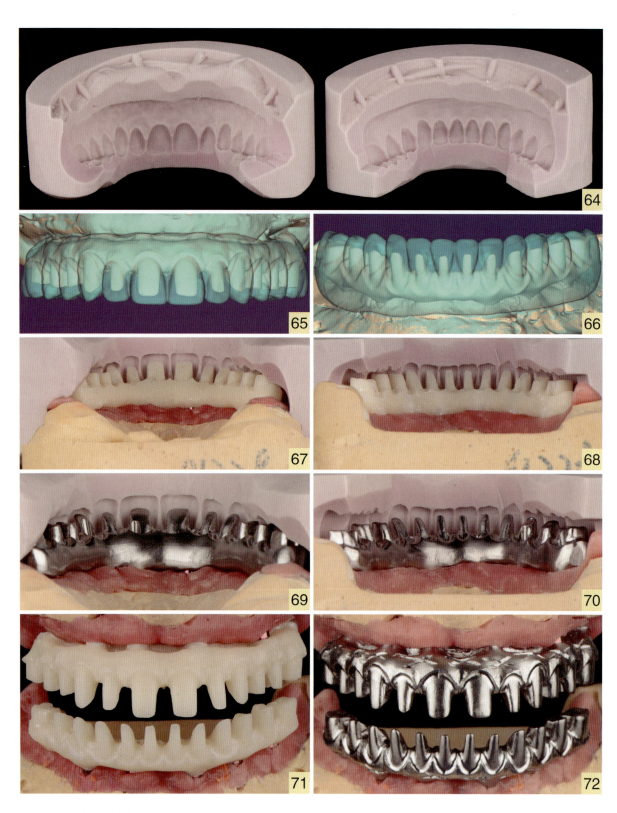

64 ~ 72 　制作钛桥架
Machined titanium frameworks

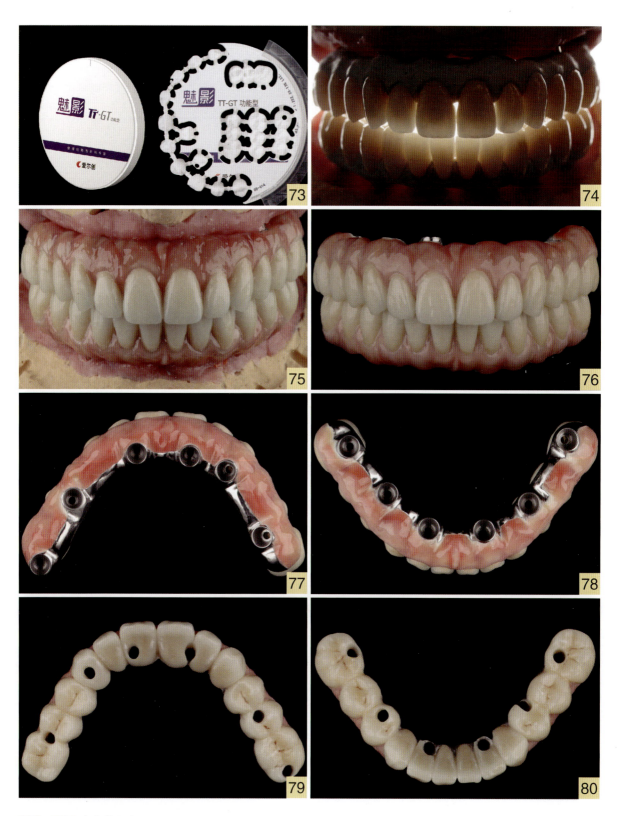

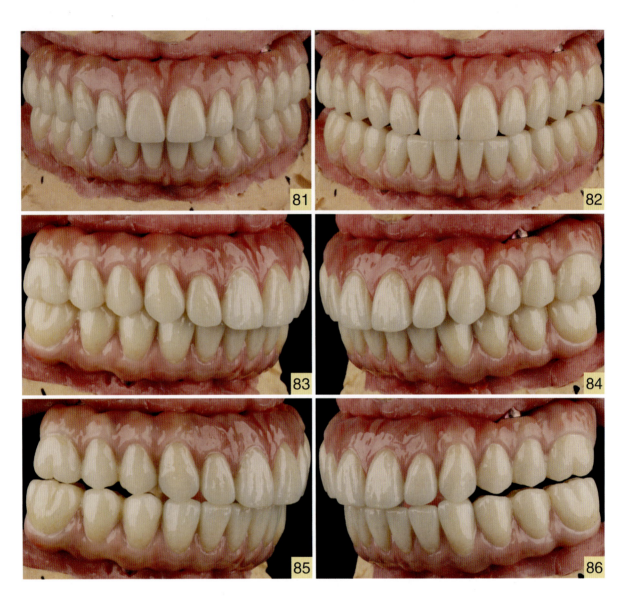

81 ~ 86 完成的义齿-2
Finished restorations-2

永久修复戴牙时取下过渡修复体，上下颌种植体稳定，牙槽黏膜未见明显红肿，口腔卫生良好（图95~图97）。将义齿于患者口内试戴，上紧二级螺丝至18Ncm（图98），并拍摄X线片确定义齿完全就位（图99）。使用聚四氟乙烯膜+流动树脂封闭螺丝孔。在患者口内调𬌗，正中𬌗双侧后牙均匀接触，前伸𬌗多颗前牙均匀接触而后牙脱离接触，侧方𬌗工作侧为组牙功能𬌗（图87~图92），再次抛光义齿，完成修复。患者获得了良好的咀嚼功能和美观效果，较治疗前有极大的改善（图93和图94）。

讨论

穿翼板种植技术难度较高，它主要应用于解决上颌磨牙区牙槽骨严重萎缩，骨量严重不足，而又希望避免大范围植骨的病例。这种技术需要医生具备高超的技能和专业的设备来确保手术的成功和患者的安全。数字化种植导板能提高种植手术的准确性，降低手术风险。本病例使用数字化种植导板，准确完成了左上磨牙区穿翼板种植体植入，实现即刻负重，术后恢复良好，最终修复效果满意。

本病例下颌牙槽嵴角化黏膜量并不宽裕。虽然下颌是全程导板引导下植入种植体，但也采用的翻瓣手术的形式。其目的就是尽量保留种植周围的角化龈组织，为种植体周围软硬组织提供更高的稳定性，保证种植治疗的长期成功。

When the transitional restorations were removed during definitive restoration delivery, the upper and lower implants were stable, the alveolar mucosa showed no obvious redness and swelling, and the oral hygiene was good (Figs. 95 to 97). The restorations were tried in the patient's mouth, the secondary screws were tightened to 18Ncm (Fig. 98), and the X-ray film was taken to confirm that the restorations were completely in place (Fig. 99). The screw holes were closed using PTFE membrane + flowable resin. In the patient's mouth, all anterior and posterior crowns functioned well in occlusion (Figs. 87 to 92). The patients obtained good masticatory function and aesthetic results, which were greatly improved compared with those before treatment (Figs. 93 and 94).

Discussion

The pterygoid plate implant technique is highly challenging and is primarily used to address severe alveolar bone resorption in the upper molar region, significant bone deficiency, and situations where extensive bone grafting is to be avoided. This technique necessitates doctors with exceptional skills and specialized equipment to ensure surgical success and patient safety. The utilization of digital implant surgical guides can enhance the precision of implant surgery and diminish surgical risks. In this instance, digital implant surgical guides were employed to precisely carry out the pterygoid plate placement in the left upper molar region, enabling immediate loading, favorable postoperative recovery, and ultimately achieving satisfactory restoration outcomes.

The amount of keratinized mucosa in the mandible in this case is limited. Despite the placement of implants in the mandible guided by a full-arch template, flap surgery was also performed. The objective was to conserve the keratinized gingival tissue surrounding the implant to the maximum extent possible, ensuring greater stability for the soft and hard tissues around the implant and guaranteeing the long-term success of implant treatment.

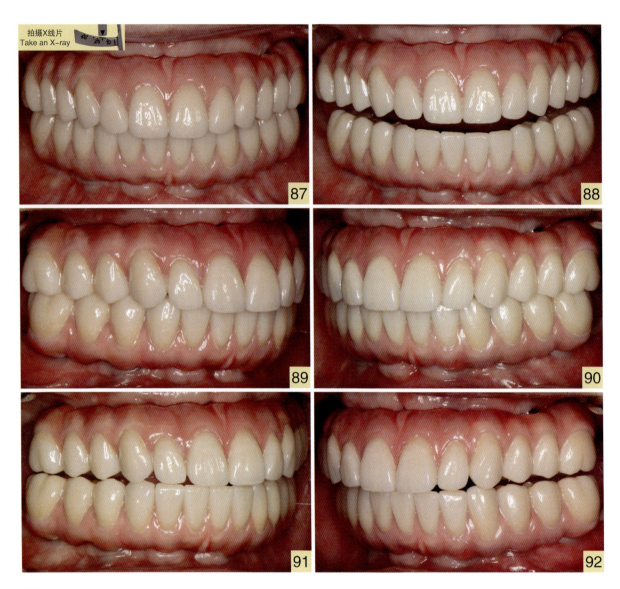

87 ~ 92 戴永久修复体-1
Delivery of the definitive restorations-1

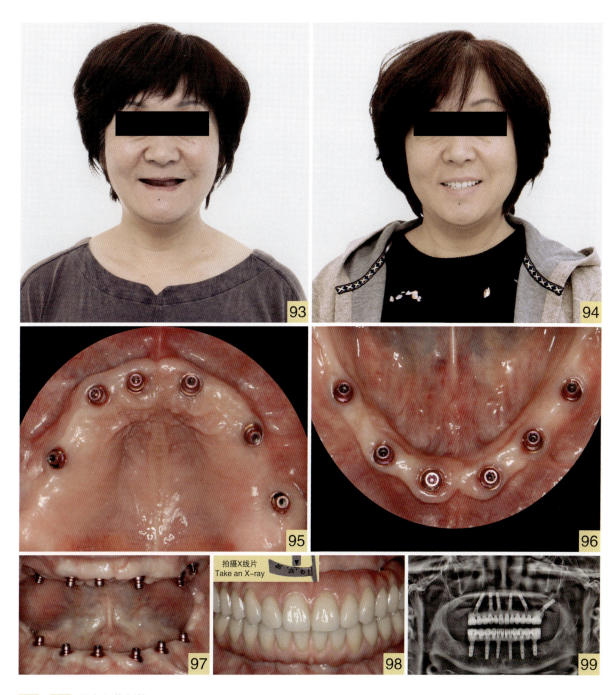

93 ~ 99 戴永久修复体-2
Delivery of the definitive restorations-2

病例7 终末期牙列黏膜支持式全程导板全口种植即刻修复一例

Case 7 Immediate Implant-supported Full-mouth Rehabilitation with Mucosal-supported Full-guided Templates for Terminal Dentitions: A Case Report

本病例资料由丁明会医生、刘海林技师提供，余涛医生整理

Provided from Dr. Minghui Ding and Dt. Hailin Liu, and arranged by Dr. Tao Yu

初诊情况

基本信息：58岁男性。

主诉：双侧上下颌前后牙缺失10余年。

现病史：10余年以来，上下颌多颗前后牙缺失，曾于外院活动义齿修复，诉戴牙不便，且近1个月余又有牙齿缺失使得义齿无法使用，现咨询种植固定修复。

既往史：无特殊。

检查：16-26、36-47缺失，牙槽骨中度至重度吸收，黏膜未见明显异常。17、27、37未见明显龋坏，叩痛（-），松动Ⅰ度，牙龈退缩，无明显红肿。上下颌位置关系基本正常，颌间距离基本合适（图2~图4）。面下1/3无明显降低，上唇丰满度略有不足（图1）。

影像学检查：曲面体层片显示上颌磨牙区剩余骨高度不足，上颌前磨牙及前牙区、下颌牙槽骨高度尚可；17、27、37牙槽骨吸收约达根长1/3，根尖周未见明显透射影（图5）。

Pretreatment

Basic information: 58-year-old male.

Chief complaint: Bilateral anterior and posterior teeth missing for more than 10 years.

History of present illness: For more than 10 years, multiple anterior and posterior teeth of the upper and lower jaws were missing, which was repaired with removable dentures in another hospital. The complaint was that it was inconvenient to wear teeth, and the dentures could not be used because of tooth loss over the past month.

Past history: No special history.

Examination: Teeth 16-26 and 36-47 were missing. The alveolar bone resorbed moderately to severely with no obvious abnormalities in the mucosa. There was no obvious caries, percussion pain or obvious redness and swelling for 17, 27 and 37. The position relationship between the upper and lower jaws was basically normal, and the intermaxillary distance was basically appropriate (Figs. 2 to 4). There was no significant reduction in the lower 1/3 of the face and a slight deficiency in the fullness of the upper lip (Fig. 1).

Radiographic examination: The height of the residual bone in the maxillary molar area was insufficient, while the height of the maxillary premolar and anterior teeth area and the mandibular alveolar bone were normal. The alveolar bone of 17, 27, 37 was absorbed up to about one-third of the root length, and no obvious radiolucency was observed around the apical region. (Fig. 5).

诊断

1. 上下颌牙列缺损。
2. 慢性牙周炎。

治疗计划

17、27、37拔除，上下颌All-on-6种植，即刻过渡修复，3个月后永久修复。

术前准备

先为患者制作了上颌放射导板，稳定颌位关系，评估美学效果（图8），并佩戴放射导板再次进行CBCT扫描。将放射导板进行光学扫描，作为制作上颌导板的数字模型，与下颌口扫、CBCT一并导入导板设计软件。

按照表1于上下颌各个位点设计植入种植体（图6和图7）。

Diagnosis

1. Maxillary and mandibular dentition defect.
2. Chronic periodontitis.

Treatment plan

Extraction of 17, 27, 37, All-on-6 implant of the upper and lower jaw, immediate transitional restoration, and permanent restoration 3 months later.

Preoperative preparation

The radiation guide plates were first made for the patient to stabilize the jaw relationship and evaluate the aesthetic effect (Fig. 8), and the patient wore them for CBCT scanning again. Optical scanning of the guide plates was used as the digital imperssion, which was imported into the guide design software together with the CBCT.

The implants were designed according to Table 1 at each site of the maxilla and mandible (Figs. 6 and 7).

表1　计划植入的种植体

牙位	种植体品牌	尺寸
16	Bredent SKY	4.5mm × 12mm
14	Bredent SKY	4.0mm × 12mm
12	Bredent SKY	3.5mm × 12mm
22	Bredent SKY	3.5mm × 12mm
24	Bredent SKY	4.0mm × 12mm
26	Bredent SKY	4.5mm × 12mm
36	Bredent SKY	4.5mm × 12mm
34	Bredent SKY	4.0mm × 12mm
32	Bredent SKY	3.5mm × 12mm
42	Bredent SKY	3.5mm × 12mm
44	Bredent SKY	4.0mm × 12mm
46	Bredent SKY	4.5mm × 12mm

Table 1　Planned implants

Tooth position	Brand of implant	Size
16	Bredent SKY	4.5×12mm
14	Bredent SKY	4.0×12mm
12	Bredent SKY	3.5×12mm
22	Bredent SKY	3.5×12mm
24	Bredent SKY	4.0×12mm
26	Bredent SKY	4.5×12mm
36	Bredent SKY	4.5×12mm
34	Bredent SKY	4.0×12mm
32	Bredent SKY	3.5×12mm
42	Bredent SKY	3.5×12mm
44	Bredent SKY	4.0×12mm
46	Bredent SKY	4.5×12mm

由于上颌磨牙区牙槽骨高度不足，16、26种植体颈部斜向远中，根尖部避开双侧上颌窦。其余种植位点牙槽骨骨量及角度尚可，均设计为直立植入种植体（图12～图23）。并于上下颌各设计4个固位钉，增加种植导板稳定性和固位力。将设计完成的导板3D打印，粘接对应的导环（图9），准备导板手术工具盒（图10）。

治疗过程

常规消毒铺巾后，17-27、37-47局部浸润麻醉，戴入上下颌种植导板，并使用硅橡胶咬合导板使之稳定，使用固位钉钻预备固位钉孔，安装固位钉固定种植导板（图11和图24），确认种植导板稳定，固位好。取下导板，上颌牙槽嵴顶切开，翻瓣（图25），再安装上颌种植导板并使用固位钉固定（图26）。因27牙冠干扰26种植备洞，故先拔除27。在种植导板引导下逐级备洞，导板引导下植入种植体（图30～图37）。种植体位置、角度良好，植入扭矩均达到45Ncm或者更高，初期稳定性良好（图27）。然后安装Fast-Fix复合基台，上紧螺丝至25Ncm（图28）。安装复合基台保护帽，并用10Ncm的扭矩旋紧（图29）。拔除17，修整并复位软组织瓣，严密缝合，上颌手术完成。

Because of insufficient alveolar bone height in the maxillary molar region, the implants of 16 and 26 were oblique distally, and the apical part avoided each maxillary sinus. The rest of the implant sites had acceptable alveolar bone mass and angle and were all designed to place the implants in an upright position (Figs. 12 to 23). Four fixation pins were designed in the upper and lower jaws respectively to increase the stability and retention force of the guided plates. The guided plates were 3D printed, the corresponding guide sleeves were bonded (Fig. 9), and the surgical toolbox of the guided plate was prepared (Fig. 10).

Treatment process

After routine disinfection and drape, local infiltration anesthesia was performed at 17-27, 37-47. The maxillary and mandibular guided plates were placed, and silicone rubber occlusal guide plate was used to make them stable. The fixation pin holes were prepared, and the fixation pins were installed to fix the guided plates (Figs. 11 and 24) to confirm that the implant guide plates were stable and retained well. After removal of the guide plate, the maxillary alveolar crest was incised and flaped (Fig. 25). Then, the maxillary implant guide plate was installed and fixed with pins (Fig. 26). Because the crown of 27 interfered 26 with the implant cavity preparation, 27 was removed first. The cavities were prepared step by step under the guidance of the implant guided plate. The implants were placed under the guidance of the guided plate (Figs. 30 to 37). The position and angle of the implant were good, the insertion torque reached 45Ncm or higher, and the initial stability was good (Fig. 27). Then, the fast-fix multi-unit abutments were installed, and the screws were tightened to 25Ncm (Fig. 28). Install the multi-unit abutment protective caps and tighten it with a torque of 10Ncm (Fig. 29). 17 was removed, the soft tissue flap was trimmed and reset, and the maxillary surgery was completed with tight suture.

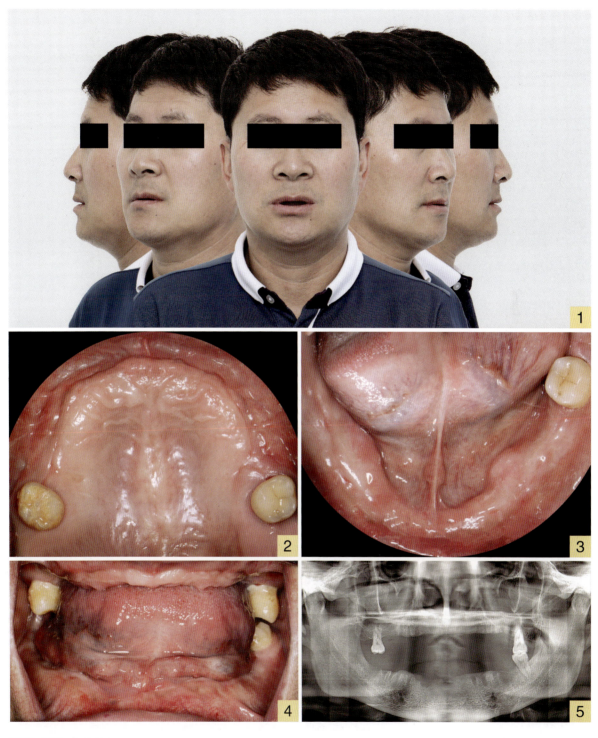

1 ~ 5　术前检查
Pretreatment examination

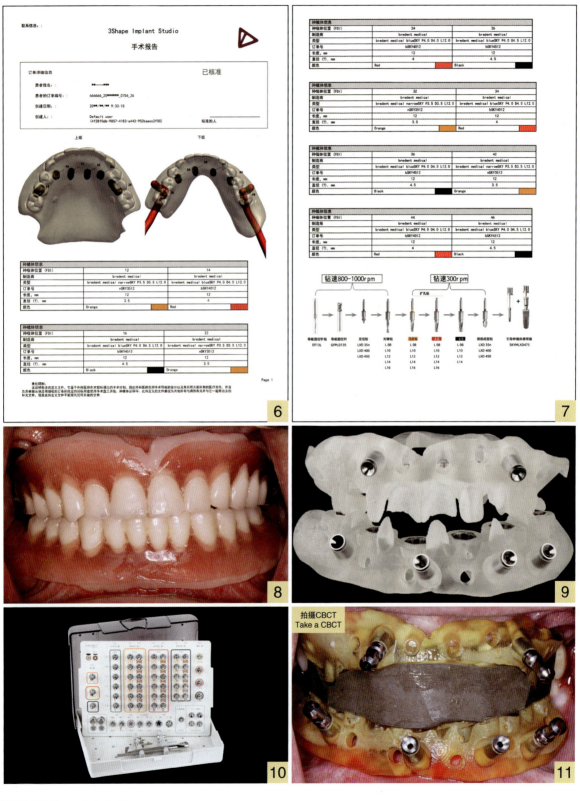

6 ~ 11　设计种植导板-1
The design of the surgical template-1

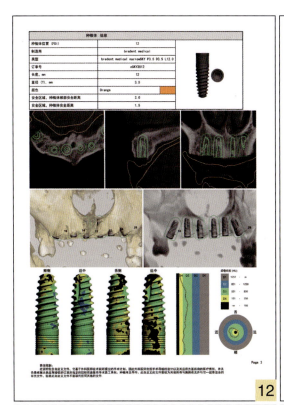

12

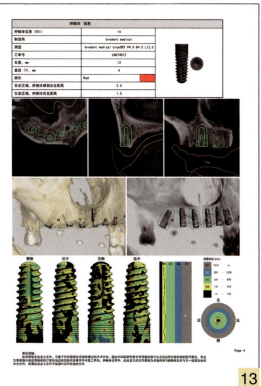

13

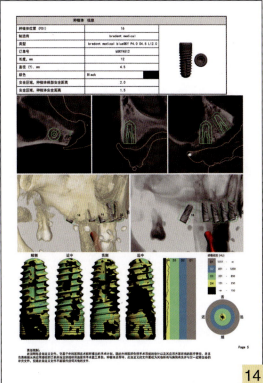

14

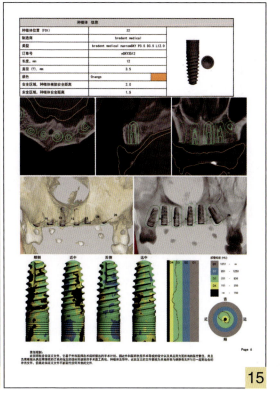

15

12 ~ 15 设计种植导板-2
The design of the surgical template-2

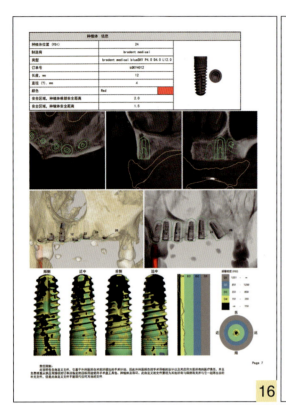

16

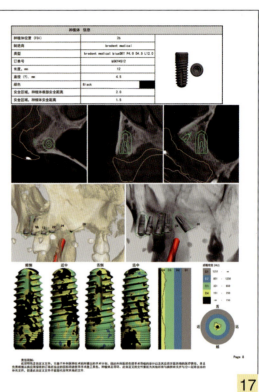

17

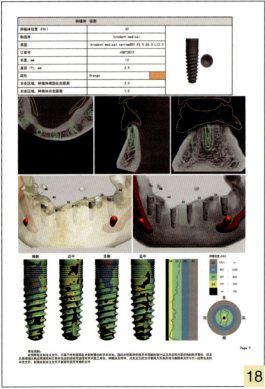

18

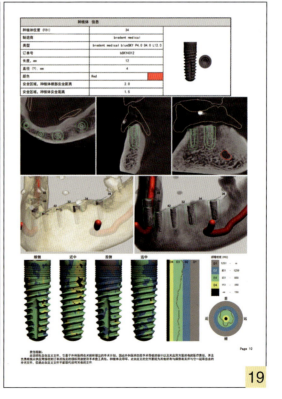

19

16 ~ 19 设计种植导板-3
The design of the surgical template-3

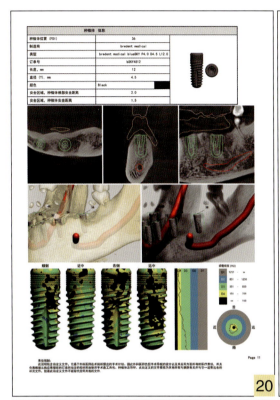

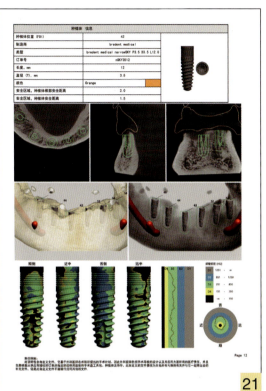

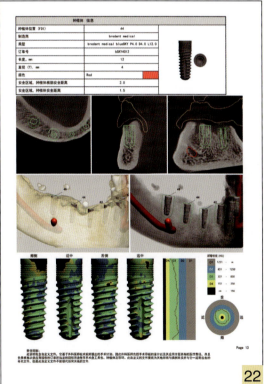

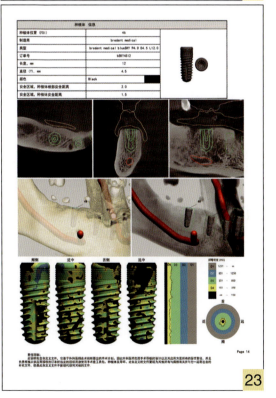

20 ~ 23 设计种植导板-4
The design of the surgical template-4

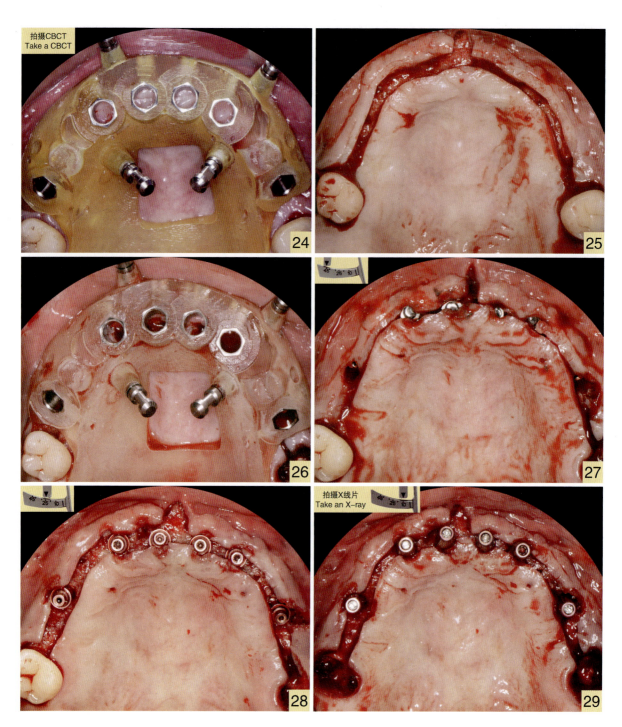

24 ~ 29 上颌术中概览
Overview of the surgery of the maxilla

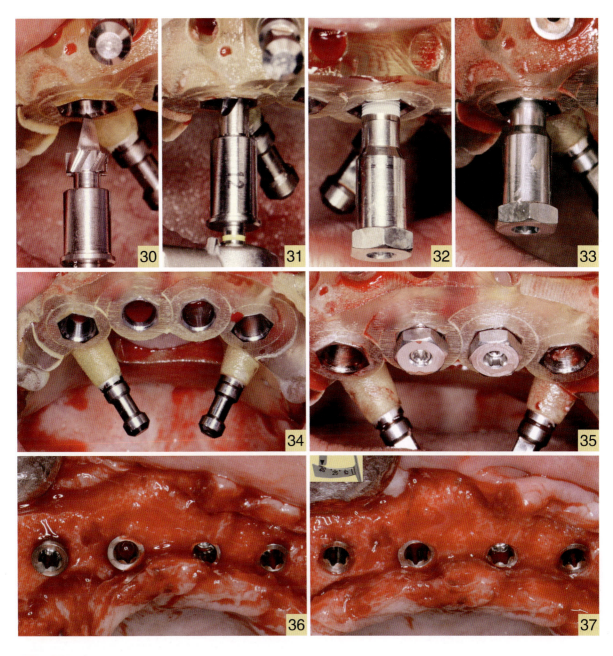

30 ~ 37 上颌术中细节
Details of the surgery of the maxilla

下颌拔除37，沿牙槽嵴顶切开，翻瓣（图39），再安装下颌种植导板并使用固位钉固定（图38）。在种植导板引导下逐级备洞（图44和图45）。导板引导下植入种植体（图46），种植体位置、角度良好，植入扭矩均达到45Ncm或者更高，初期稳定性良好（图40）。由于部分种植体颈部位于骨下，可能会干扰复合基台就位，故而安装封闭螺丝并修整牙槽骨（图41和图47），之后再取下封闭螺丝，便能够顺利安装Fast-Fix复合基台，上紧螺丝至25Ncm（图42和图48）。安装复合基台保护帽，并用10Ncm的扭矩旋紧（图43）。修整并复位软组织瓣，严密缝合，下颌手术完成（图52）。

拍片确认所有种植体位置良好，复合基台完全就位后，使用硅橡胶制取颌位记录，确定中线、𬌗平面。取下复合基台保护帽，安装复合基台水平转移杆，拍片确认转移杆完全就位，再使用牙科种植用连接件+成型树脂在口内连接，上下颌均使用硅橡胶制取开窗夹板式基台水平印模。再次安装复合基台保护帽。将印模转至技工室灌模型，上𬌗架，制作即刻过渡义齿。并于手术当天取下复合基台保护帽，为患者戴入即刻过渡义齿，二级螺丝旋紧至18Ncm（图50、图51和图53），拍片确认义齿完全就位（图54），即刻为患者恢复咀嚼功能，改善牙齿美观（图49）。

For the mandible, 37 was extracted and the alveolar ridge was incised and flapped (Fig. 39). Then the mandibular guided plate again installed and fixed using fixation pins (Fig. 38). The holes were prepared step by step under the guidance of the guided plate (Figs. 44 and 45). The implants were placed under the guidance of the guide plate (Fig. 46), and the implant position and angle were good. The insertion torque reached 45Ncm or higher, and the initial stability was good (Fig. 40). Because some of the implant neck is located under the bone, it may interfere with the placement of the multi-unit abutments. Therefore, the sealing screws were installed and the alveolar bone was trimmed (Figs. 41 and 47). After removing the sealing screws, the fast-fix multi-unit abutments could be successfully installed, and the screws were tight to 25Ncm (Figs. 42 and 48). Install the multi-unit abutments protective cap and tighten it with a torque of 10Ncm (Fig. 43). The soft tissue flap was trimmed and reset, tightly sutured, and the mandibular surgery was completed (Fig. 52).

Radiographs were taken to confirm that all implants were in good position and the multi-unit abutments were completely in place. Silicone rubber was used to record the jaw position and determine the midline and occlusal plane. The protective caps of the multi-unit abutments were removed, and the transfer copings of the multi-unit abutments were installed. The X-ray film was taken to confirm that the transfer copings were completely in place, then the steel pods and pattern resin were used to connect the transfer copings in the mouth. Install the multi-unit abutments protective caps again. The occlusal records and the impressions were sent to the lab to fabricate the immediate interim restorations in a rapid way. On the day of surgery, the protective caps of the multi-unit abutments were removed, and the immediate interim restorations were delivered. The secondary screws were tightened to 18Ncm (Figs. 50, 51, and 53), and the restorations were confirmed to be completely in place (Fig. 54). The masticatory function and esthetic appearance were regained (Fig. 49).

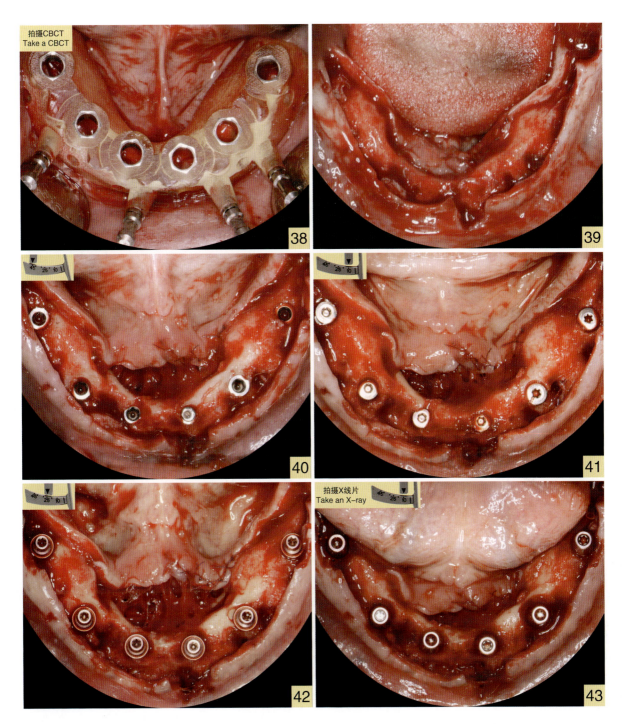

38 ~ 43 下颌术中概览
Overview of the surgery of the mandibular

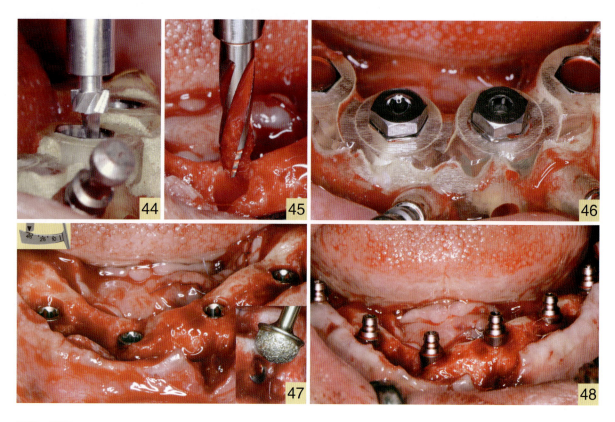

44 ~ 48 下颌术中细节
Details of the surgery of the mandibular

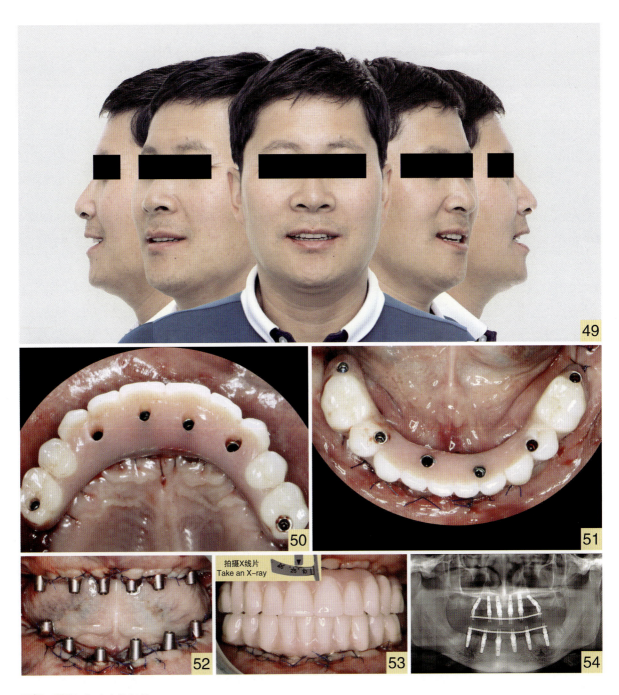

49 ~ 54 戴过渡修复体
Delivery of the immediate restorations

蜕变——数字化种植导板与全瓷修复中的医技实践
Metamorphosis: Clinical and Technological Practices in Digital Surgical Templates and Ceramic Restorations for Implants

过渡修复3个月后，患者无不适主诉，对过渡修复效果较为满意，检查发现过渡义齿稳定，种植体无松动（图55），拍摄曲面体层片显示种植体周围牙槽骨稳定，未见明显低密度影（图57）。取下过渡义齿，将所有复合基台再次加力至25Ncm，安装复合基台转移杆并用成型树脂于口内再次连接，使用个别托盘制取上下颌硅橡胶开窗夹板式基台水平印模，灌制石膏模型，用过渡义齿与硅橡胶制取咬合记录并将模型上𬌗架。为患者制作评估桥，戴入口内后拍片确认完全就位（图58），评估桥中线、𬌗平面正确，前牙丰满度合适，垂直距离合适，正中关系正确，双侧咬合均匀稳定，患者对牙齿排列满意（图56）。

光学扫描评估桥并数字化复制其外形，回切全瓷牙冠及牙龈部分烤塑空间（图59和图60）。切削正式钛架，并确认全瓷牙冠修复及牙龈部分烤塑空间合适（图62）。钛架表面遮色（图61），光学扫描，设计16-26、36-46全瓷冠，并用高透渐变色氧化锆制作全冠（图63）。牙冠唇颊侧少量烤瓷，染色，上釉（图64和图65）；牙龈部分进行烤塑，模拟天然牙龈颜色（图66）。义齿表面高度抛光，并在组织面留出牙缝刷清洁通道（图67～图71）。义齿再上𬌗架进行调𬌗，抛光（图72～图77）。

After 3 months, the patient had no complaints of discomfort and was satisfied with the effect of the transitional restorations. The examination showed that the transitional restorations were stable, and the implants were not loose (Fig. 55). Panoramic tomography showed that the alveolar bone around the implants was stable and no obvious low-density shadow was found (Fig. 57). After the transition restorations were removed, all the multi-unit abutments were re-forced to 25Ncm, and the multi-unit abutment transfer copings were installed and re-connected with pattern resin in the mouth. The impressions of the upper and lower jaw were made with silicone rubber using individual trays, and the plaster casts were poured. Evaluation bridges were made for the patient, and radiographs were taken to confirm that the bridges were completely in place (Fig. 58). It was evaluated that the middle line and occlusal plane of the bridge were correct, the fullness of the anterior teeth was appropriate, the vertical distance was appropriate, the centric relationship was correct, the bilateral occlusion was uniform and stable, and the patient was satisfied with the arrangement of the teeth (Fig. 56).

The evaluation bridges were optical scanned. Cut back was performed to achieve enough spaces for all ceramic crowns and plastic gingiva (Figs. 59 and 60). Titanium frameworks were machined and confirmed to have appropriate space for the full ceramic crown restorations and the gum part baking plastic space are appropriate (Fig. 62). The surface of the titanium frame was opaque (Fig. 61) and optical scanned. 16-26 and 36-46 all ceramic crowns were designed and produced by high transparent zirconia (Fig. 63). A small amount of porcelain on the buccal side of the crown was stained and glazed (Figs. 64 and 65). The gum part was baked with plastic to mimic the natural gum color (Fig. 66). The surfaces of the restorations were highly polished, and interdental brush cleaning channels were left on the tissue surfaces (Figs. 67 to 71). The restorations were then put on the articulator for occlusal adjustment and were then polished (Figs. 72 to 77).

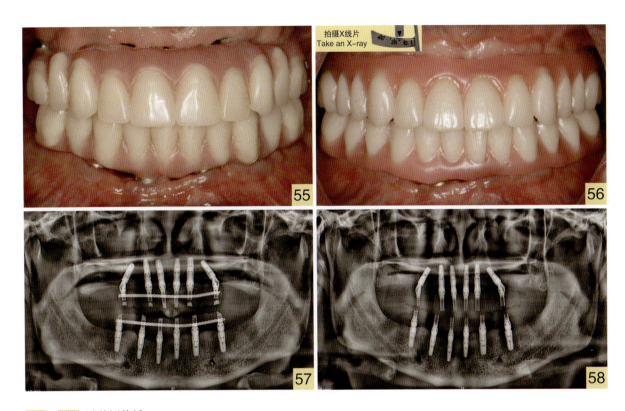

55~58 试戴评估桥
Try-in of evaluation bridge

永久修复戴牙时取下过渡修复体，上下颌种植体稳定，牙槽黏膜未见明显红肿，口腔卫生良好（图78、图79和图82）。将义齿于患者口内试戴，上紧二级螺丝至18Ncm（图83），并拍摄X线片确定义齿完全就位（图84）。使用聚四氟乙烯膜+流动树脂封闭螺丝孔，在患者口内调粭，抛光，完成修复（图80、图81、图85~图90）。患者获得了良好的咀嚼功能和美观效果，对治疗效果较为满意（图91~图94）。

When the transitional restorations were removed, the upper and lower implants were stable, the alveolar mucosa showed no obvious redness and swelling, and the oral hygiene was good (Figs. 78, 79, and 82). The restorations were tried in the patient's mouth, the secondary screws were tightened to 18Ncm (Fig. 83), and the X-ray film was taken to confirm that the restorations were completely in place (Fig. 84). The screw holes were closed with PTFE membrane + flowable resin, adjusted and polished in the patient's mouth to complete the restoration (Figs. 80, 81, 85 to 90). The patient obtained good masticatory function and aesthetic results and was satisfied with the treatment results (Figs. 91 to 94).

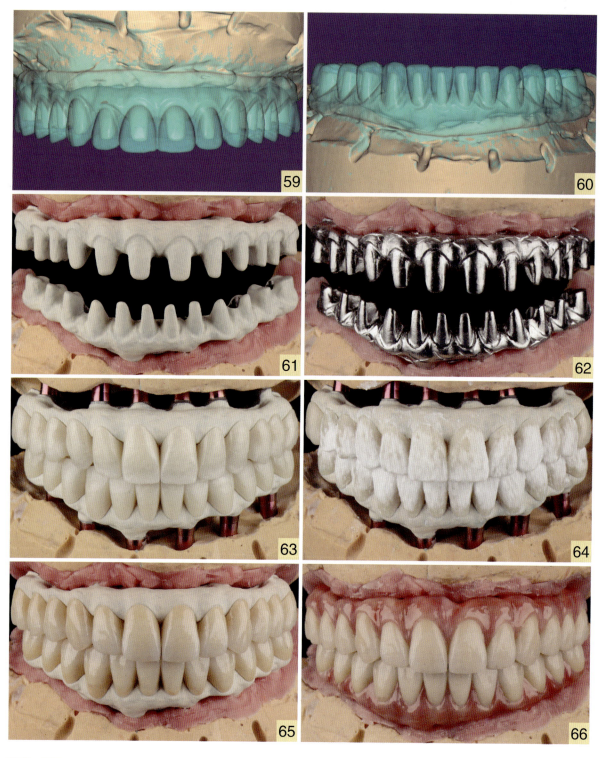

59 ~ 66 制作钛桥架
Machined titanium frameworks

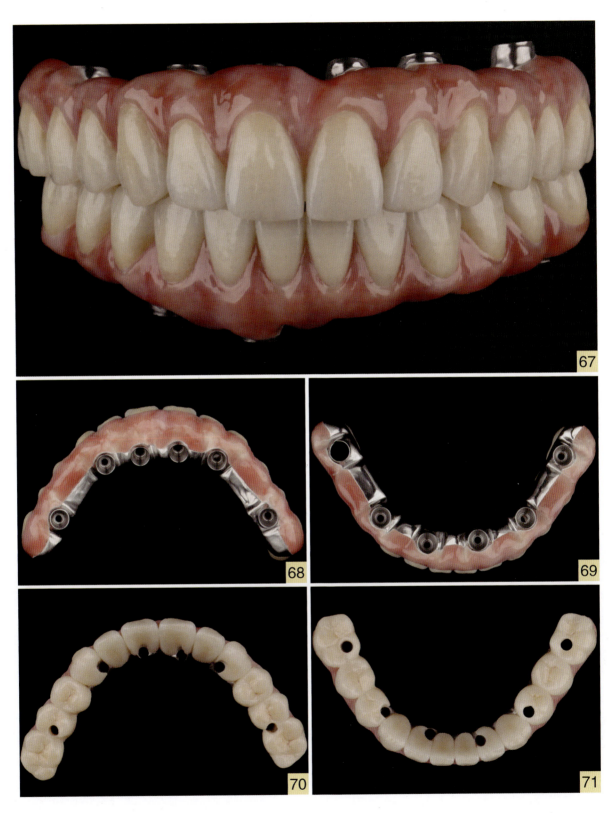

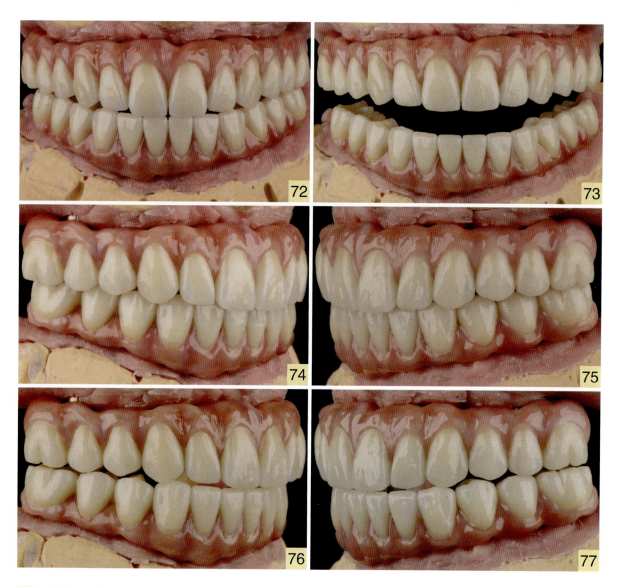

72 ~ 77 完成的义齿-2
Finished restorations-2

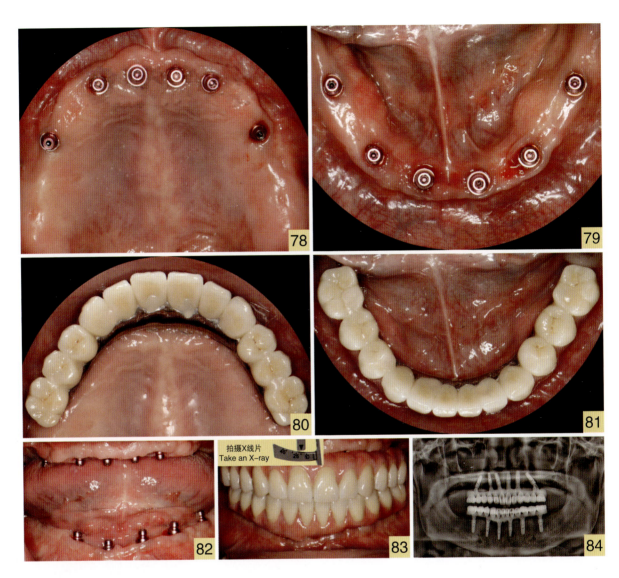

拍摄X线片
Take an X-ray

78 ~ 84 戴永久修复体–1
Delivery of the definitive restorations-1

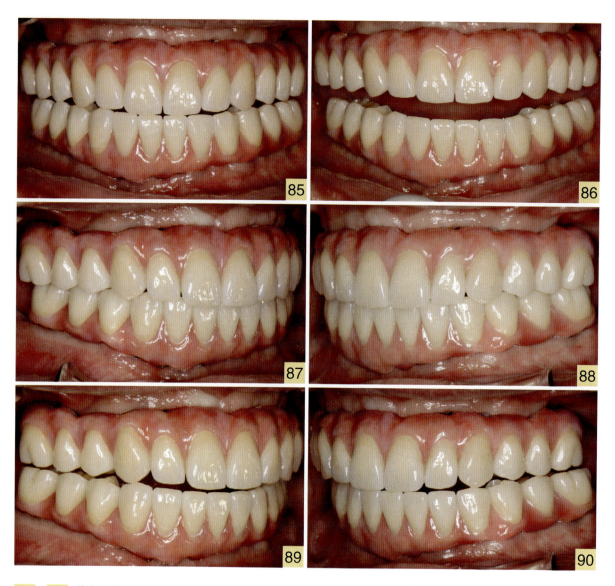

85 ~ 90 戴永久修复体-2
Delivery of the definitive restorations-2

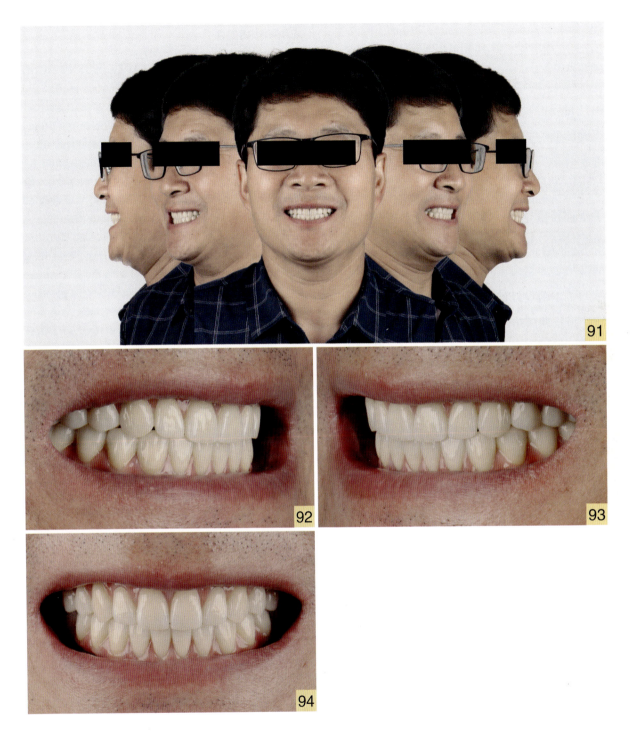

91 ~ 94　戴永久修复体–3
Delivery of the definitive restorations-3